IronFit®
Strength Training
and Nutrition
for Endurance Athletes

Also by Don Fink

Be Iron Fit: Time-Efficient Training Secrets for Ultimate Fitness
Mastering the Marathon: Time-Efficient Training Secrets for the 40-plus Athlete

IronFit®

Strength Training and Nutrition for Endurance Athletes

Time-Efficient Training Secrets for Breakthrough Fitness

Don Fink and Melanie Fink

LYONS PRESS
Guilford, Connecticut
An imprint of Globe Pequot Press

Lyons Press is an imprint of Globe Pequot Press

Ironman and Ironman Triathlon are registered trademarks of the World Triathlon Corporation

IronFit is a registered trademark of Don Fink

All exercise technique photos featuring Yvonne Hernandez are provided courtesy of Lynn Kellogg/www.trilifephotos.com.

Text design and layout: Mary Ballachino
Project editor: Ellen Urban

Library of Congress Cataloging-in-Publication Data is available on file.

ISBN 978-0-7627-8294-9

Printed in the United States of America

10 9 8 7 6 5 4 3 2 1

MEDICAL DISCLAIMER

The programs in this book are designed for athletes with either a high level of fitness or the physiology to attain a high level of fitness. Readers should consult a physician before beginning any of the workouts suggested herein. If you experience any pain or difficulty with these exercises, stop and consult your health-care provider.

To our loving parents,
Esther and Martin and Claire and Richard

Contents

Introduction

Strength training and nutrition—they go hand in hand. It's not always easy to see the relationship, but in addition to the sport-specific training of an endurance athlete (the actual running, cycling, swimming, etc.), the proper combination of strength training and nutrition can make the difference between merely improving and breaking through to entirely new levels of competitive performance.

When we say *strength training*, we are referring not only to traditional weight lifting at the gym; we're also talking about core and functional strength training—about developing core muscles and muscle/movement balance, as well as enhancing each of the movements specific to an athlete's sport.

When we say *nutrition*, we are not just talking about what a person eats and drinks each day, although this is important, and we'll discuss it in great detail. We are also talking about what we eat and drink before, during, and after training sessions and competitions to prepare our bodies to perform at our highest levels, and to recover healthily after great exertion.

This book will help any athlete who is training and competing in any endurance event or sport. By adding the proper strength-training program and nutritional approach, any good sport-specific training plan can be converted into something truly amazing. The programs in this book are designed to work especially well with our triathlon-specific training programs in *Be Iron Fit*, and our marathon-specific programs in *Mastering the Marathon*, but they can also be used with any sport-specific program an athlete has undertaken to create truly exceptional training.

This book is divided into nine major sections—Chapters 1 through 9—four of which are packed with actual programs and routines that an athlete can put into action to derive immediate benefits.

First, we discuss strength training and how we can properly use it to build functional strength and muscle/movement balance crucial to endurance sports athletes while also using it to make us less injury-prone. We will move beyond the traditional strength-training approaches of static machines to examine the new cutting-edge approaches to building functional, dynamic, and sport-specific strength and power. While we may still use some traditional equipment like dumbbells, we will approach their use with a focus on functional training. We will combine traditional equipment with the use of the stability ball (Swiss ball), foam roller, BOSU ball, and other effective functional strength- and core-training equipment.

This book details nine specific strength-training programs, each tailored to different types of endurance athletes. While each of the programs has similar philosophies and approaches, they are built upon the principle that different sports require different focuses. The nine programs presented here each focus on a particular sport with progressions for each exercise. The athlete may begin at the basic level, and as he or she gets stronger, each exercise offers up to two progressions.

In addition to the nine sport-specific strength-training programs, this book also offers several special programs to further enhance an athlete's training. These include efficient warm-up and stretching routines that can be used with any of the strength and core programs. Breathing and mental exercises are described to help the athlete get centered and focused for the challenge ahead. We even include a special travel program for the athlete who is traveling without access to gym facilities. This program can be done in a hotel room and requires little to no equipment.

Each strength program is designed to be time-efficient, effective, and fun. Busy athletes training for endurance sports don't have the time for long, complicated, and often boring workouts. Each workout in this book is fine-tuned to ten or fewer time-efficient, fun, and results-oriented exercises.

In Chapter 4, we move from strength training to a discussion about nutrition. We describe what an athlete needs to eat and drink before, during, and after training and competition, as well as how an athlete should approach day-to-day nutrition for best results.

We will discuss overall healthy eating for endurance athletes, presenting our approach to six small daily meals, and we will explain how to balance these meals properly between proteins, fats, and carbohydrates, while keeping overall calorie consumption in mind. We will also provide tools to help athletes determine how many calories should be consumed each day to achieve and maintain optimal race weight.

The next chapter presents five complete seven-day healthy eating plans. Using daily calorie targets and other factors, we explain how the athlete will select the plan that fits him or her best. From here, the athlete will learn how to make ongoing substitutions to the seven-day regimen to create a healthy eating plan for life.

Following nutrition, we discuss the crucial topic of hydration. We will explain hydration's great importance and the impact it has on our performance, and also present the tools athletes can use to precisely determine their unique hydration needs, no matter the race and the conditions. We discuss the logistics of hydration and how to develop a personalized hydration routine.

We then tackle the subject of what we like to call "fueling." Chapter 7 provides our specific nutritional plan to be used before, during, and after training and competition. The information in this chapter allows athletes to determine their own unique optimal fueling requirements, along with racing logistics and other needs.

Finally, we offer complete fueling and hydration plans for eight experienced and accomplished endurance athletes. These plans include exactly what the competitors eat and drink before, during, and after both training and racing for best results. In addition to these successful battle-tested plans, we present the tools needed to fine-tune these plans to perfectly fit each athlete.

The premise of this book is that to achieve your optimal level of performance in a sport, much more is required than what meets the eye. Simply training in a sport is not enough to get you there. Runners cannot obtain their most competitive performance level merely by running; likewise, cyclists cannot reach their most competitive performance level merely by cycling, and swimmers, merely by swimming. No matter how good your sport-specific training, your athletic performance can be taken to an entirely new level by complementing a training program with the proper strength training, race and training nutrition, and an overall healthy eating plan. This book empowers you—the triathlete, the duathlete, the runner, the cyclist, the swimmer—to do exactly that.

So, let's turn the page and get started building your endurance sports performance to an entirely new level!

CHAPTER 1

The Power of Functional Strength and Core Training

The perfect is the enemy of the good.

—Voltaire

When the running boom first hit the United States in the 1970s, virtually no connection existed between strength training and endurance sports. It was as if endurance sports sat on the opposite end of the sports spectrum from "muscle sports"—night-and-day endeavors.

The Evolution of Strength Training in Endurance Sports

Coauthor Don remembers when, as a high school cross-country runner, strength training of any type was pretty much frowned upon by his coaches, if not openly discouraged. "You will bulk up with big muscles and that will slow you down" was the general philosophy of the time.

But over the years the exclusion of strength training from endurance sports gradually diminished. We first started to see strength training being used by endurance athletes in the context of rehabilitation from injury. Trainers and physical therapists helped athletes build back from injury using specific types of strength-training exercises.

This trend evolved into using strength training as a way not only to recover from injury, but also to help prevent injury in the first place. Experts developed a much greater appreciation of how sports can create muscle/movement imbalances over time. While the athlete is building certain types of muscle strength through his or her sport, often other areas are gradually becoming comparatively weaker. These imbalances can contribute to injury.

Take, for example, the sport of swimming. As an athlete builds shoulder and upper-back muscles through swimming, the chest and other areas become comparatively weaker. Some swimmers even develop an exaggerated, rounded shoulder look as a result. These types of muscle imbalances

1

can lead to structural and postural misalignments, which can cause undue stress and eventual acute-type injuries to tendons, ligaments, and joints.

The sports world's progressive appreciation of strength training to correct imbalances can be seen in coauthor Melanie's athletic history. Melanie was continually frustrated by knee pain throughout her twenties and early thirties. It seemed that as soon as she would train herself into great form and start to race at her very best, the knee pain would return. Year after year she would end up seeing a sports doctor who would diagnose patellar tendonitis and recommend that she rest. Nothing is as frustrating to an athlete who has successfully trained into great form than being told to stop. All you can think about is how quickly your hard-earned fitness will slip away and how long it will take to get back to previous levels.

What we didn't understand at the time was that as Melanie built up her training volume, muscle imbalances were being created in her body that led to her knee pain. The simplest explanation is that the muscles of her hamstring group were weaker than her quadriceps femoris group, which gets a heavy workload during the act of running. When the stronger quads flexed to extend the knee, the weaker hamstring was unable to prevent friction and inflammation in the tendon that connects the kneecap to the shin. The result: It became difficult and painful to run and walk. But, as we'll explain further, muscle balance is a bigger-picture idea.

As the years passed, some doctors recommended physical therapy in addition to rest. This prescription was a step in the right direction, but the traditional strength-training exercises remained focused on building the muscles just around the knee itself—quads and hamstrings. Melanie would do these exercises faithfully and build up these muscles, but as soon as she built her training volume back up, the pain would return.

Melanie finally discovered the solution to her challenge in her late thirties. Fortunately, she found a forward-thinking trainer who showed her how, through proper functional strength training, she could correct these imbalances and become more injury-proof. The problem was that while traditional strength-training exercises helped to build specific strength in the weaker muscles around the knee, they did not build the kind of functional strength required by a competitive athlete. While the pain symptoms occurred in the knee, the cause of the pain came from muscle imbalances throughout her body—all the body's muscles involved in the system of force and stabilization that results in a properly bent and extended knee.

2

It has now been several years since Melanie started training for muscle/movement balance, and happily, her knee pain is a thing of the past. In fact, after so many years of her recurring knee issue, we realized that she had not mentioned it in ages.

To really make the point, Melanie recently trained for an entire year to compete in the Ultraman Canada competition in Penticton, British Columbia. This event includes a 6.2-mile open-water swim followed by 260 miles of cycling, and then a 52.4-mile double marathon. Melanie stuck with her functional strength and core training throughout her many months of swim, bike, and run training, just as she has for the past ten-plus years, right up until her pre-race taper. Amazingly, she didn't endure knee pain once. She covered all those miles, including a double marathon at the end, and her knees were completely free of pain.

The most recent phase in the evolution of endurance-sport strength came when we began to see the use of strength training move from merely correcting imbalances to a focus on actually developing sport-specific functional strength.

We have finally arrived with functional strength training.

It took us a while to get here, but this strength-training philosophy is where we always needed to be. Not only will we use functional strength training to correct muscle imbalances and build sport-specific strength, but we will also build a different kind of strength. It will be a dynamic strength directly related to the biomechanical movements needed for each individual sport.

The programs presented in this book are designed to help the athlete select the optimal strength-training program for his or her specific sport, along with the specific athletic movements. While there are many similarities among endurance sports, there are also important subtle differences that, if taken into account, will make an athlete's preparation significantly better.

Oh, yeah; one more point: You are going to love functional strength training. It's addictive. When Don was first introduced to functional strength training years ago, he described long-dormant muscles springing back to life. His balance, agility, and functional movement improved almost immediately. From now on, you will look forward to your strength-training days like never before.

The Core Muscles

A major part of the progression of strength training in endurance sports over the past few decades lies in how we view the role of our core muscles. By core muscles, we mean all the muscles in the body's middle area, especially the abdominals, back, buttocks, pelvic floor, and hips.

Until recent years, this area was at best given little consideration, and at worst, overlooked altogether. The focus of strength training was traditionally on exercises for the arms, shoulders, chest, and legs. Perhaps some sit-ups or crunches were thrown in at the end of a strength program to work on the abdominals, but even then, the focus was on the appearance of the abdominals rather than their function.

The most common exercise most athletes would do for the abdominals was crunches. This exercise begins in a lying position on the floor; knees are bent, and hands are behind the athlete's head. The athlete then pulls his head and elbows toward his knees to complete the crunch. Ironically, what this popular exercise actually does is shorten the abdominals and limit them functionally. When performing most endurance sports, we need to elongate our muscles, not shorten them. Think about reaching, extending, twisting, pulling, etc.

Since the days of "do some crunches," it has become more generally understood that the core muscles are not only more important than previously realized, but in fact may be the most important of all. In addition to helping to stabilize the spine, the core is involved in virtually all athletic movement. No matter how much stronger you become in your arms, shoulders, chest, and legs, if your core is weak, it will not only greatly reduce your athletic ability, but it will also likely increase your risk for injury. The core muscles promote proper functioning of the other muscles along with proper power transfer to the arms and legs.

Just try to think of any athletic movement you can do without involving the core muscles. Running, jumping, throwing, kicking, pushing, pulling, you name it—it involves the core muscles. In fact, most simple nonathletic movements involve the core, as well. Just try to get out of bed in the morning without engaging your abdominals. Then try to take your first step of the day without engaging your gluteus. You can't do it. The core muscles are that critical to even the simplest of our moments.

The acceptance of core training's importance for endurance athletes has been a long time coming. Even today we encounter athletes who consider themselves "old school" and want to stick to traditional weight lifting, no matter what. To them, strength training means weights and machines, not an exercise ball, stretch cords, and a BOSU. We even know a fifty-something-year-old triathlete who insists on using a free-weights squat rack with more than two times his body weight because he thinks it will improve his cycling power. All we can say is that we hope he has good medical insurance.

The results are clear: Combining proper functional strength and core training with endurance training can greatly improve an athlete's speed, balance, and sport-specific strength, while also helping him or her to be more injury-resistant.

Sean Reilly, a regular competitor at the Ironman World Championships in Kona, Hawaii, credits proper core and functional strength training for keeping him competing at an elite level into his forties. "As I've gotten older," he says, "strength training has helped me to stay injury-free throughout the season."

Muscle: Use It or Lose It

In addition to the aforementioned reasons for endurance athletes to properly include sport-specific functional strength and core training into an overall training program, another very important motivation exists for athletes and nonathletes alike to make regular functional strength and core training part of their lives: age-related muscle loss.

According to the American Council on Exercise, after the age of twenty-five, we lose approximately a half-pound of lean muscle per year. This condition is generally referred to as *sarcopenia*.

Many athletes mistakenly believe that as long as they are active, they will continue to maintain and build muscle. Unfortunately, this is not the case, especially with endurance sports athletes. While endurance sports may help to reduce the negative effects of sarcopenia, endurance sports alone are not enough to get the job done. Only proper strength training will prevent or even reverse the effects of age-related muscle loss.

Time Management of Strength and Core Training

Having coached hundreds of athletes over many years, we find that while there are some who simply do not accept or understand the importance of functional strength and core training, there are others who neglect it simply because it takes time. Strength training gets squeezed out as the season goes on and an athlete's overall training hours increase.

We often see athletes start the year with a great strength and core program, but as the training hours increase, they find that they either don't have the time to fit in their strength training or they are just too tired from all the other training to get through a long program. We see this again and again.

Take the case of Iron-distance triathlete "John Irontri." In the off-season, he trains fewer than ten hours per week and can easily find time for two or even three one-hour strength and core sessions. But endurance athletes are like everyone else. They have families, careers, and many other responsibilities. As the season progresses and Mr. Irontri's swim, bike, and run training time creep up to as much as twenty hours per week, he finds he can no longer find the time for two one-hour strength-training sessions, or honestly, even if he could, he doesn't have the desire. After a long five- to six-hour bike ride or a two- to three-hour run, who really wants to strength-train for an hour?

The solution is a somewhat-controversial one (and we know many "by-the-book" personal trainers reading this section are going to gasp at our blasphemy): shorter, more-efficient strength- and core-training programs. While two to three 45- to 60-minute programs per week can be completed during the off-season, when we get to the preseason and competitive season, it becomes increasingly tough to fit even two of these sessions in per week, let alone have the energy to do them. What we have found from working with hundreds of busy athletes for many years is that strength-and-core neglect is not the case with a very efficient 20- to 30-minute program.

In addition to the obvious—that it's easier to find 20 to 30 minutes than 60 minutes in a busy schedule—it's also mentally easier to persuade yourself to do a shorter program when you are already feeling a bit tired, or even overwhelmed by your training. When you arrive back home after a five- to six-hour training ride, it's a real challenge to talk yourself (not to mention your spouse) into now completing a 60-minute strength-training program. But a 20- to 30-minute program? That's a different story. In fact, many of our coached athletes have told us that if they just get going on it and don't stress about it too much, it's over before they know it.

What we have come to realize is expressed in the famous Voltaire quote: "The perfect is the enemy of the good." If we insist on an absolutely complete and thorough program that covers everything as perfectly as possible, chances are it won't get done. No matter how perfect the program, it's worthless if nobody does it. If the athlete finds it to be too long to fit into his or her overall schedule, given constraints on time and energy, then it's of no use.

The solution is to design programs that are very efficient, that complement the athlete's sport-specific training, and that can still be consistently completed, even when the athlete's time and energy pressures increase. While the program may not hit every single exercise that it might include in a perfect world, it gives the athlete what he needs in a short-enough form so that he can find the time and energy to complete it consistently.

The programs presented in Chapters 2 and 3 are designed with this approach in mind. They are designed to be fun, productive, and time-efficient. Most important, they are proven. They are "battlefield-tested" by busy endurance athletes, with great results.

Frequency, Timing, and Training Cycles

Successful strength training, like all training, relies on the "overload principle." The American Council on Exercise defines this as "One of the principles of human performance that states that beneficial adaptations occur in response to demands applied to the body at levels beyond a certain threshold (overload), but within the limits of tolerance and safety." In simple terms, our bodies either need to work harder or in a different way than they are used to working in order to improve.

If we do the exact same 3-mile run at the same pace three times per week, we will eventually hit a plateau and our fitness and performance will no longer improve. In fact, it will become stagnant and eventually probably even decline. Likewise, if we do the exact same strength-training routine with the same weights and number of sets and repetitions week after week, we will plateau and our fitness and performance will no longer improve.

We need to introduce gradual "overloads" to our training to stimulate improvement. We include the word gradual because this kind of training will only work if the proper amount of overload is introduced. If it's too much of an overload, it can cause a breakdown, and no improvement will be gained. Conversely, if it's too modest of an overload, it will not be enough to stimulate growth. The overload needs to be just the right amount to stimulate the fitness improvements we want. The programs presented in this book are designed to do exactly that.

In general, we suggest a frequency of strength and core training for endurance athletes of one to three times per week on nonconsecutive days year-round. It's important to strength-train consistently to prevent and reverse the effects of age-related muscle loss. Whether or not you are a competitive athlete, strength exercises are something we should all be doing at some level all of the time.

As you will see in the functional strength- and core-training programs presented in this book, we suggest that athletes approach their strength training in three cycles throughout the year: Off-Season, Preseason, and Competitive Season. As the athlete's training progresses through phases—as we show in our other training books, *Be Iron Fit* and *Mastering the Marathon*—strength- and core-training programs need to progress through cycles as well.

In the Off-Season, we will focus on building our base functional strength for our sport. Then, in the Preseason, before our bodies become too comfortable with our exercises, we will graduate to higher progression levels and dynamic movements and add some new exercises. These subtle changes are just what we need to stimulate further development and improvement in our functional strength and power. Finally, once we are into our Competitive Season, the exercises will change again as our focus shifts to maintaining functional strength and avoiding injury.

The frequency of one to three strength-training sessions per week

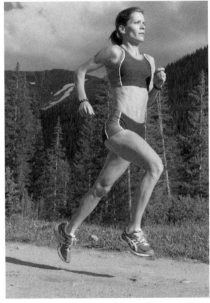

World-class marathoner Adriana Nelson
Photo courtesy of 101 Degrees West

8

may vary based on the specific athlete's situation and goals, but it is a suitable range for most. Two times per week is enough for the vast majority, especially once they are into the preseason and competitive season. If an athlete wants to train three times per week, that's absolutely fine. Typically, we suggest that most athletes do two to three sessions in the Off-Season, two sessions in the Preseason, and one to two sessions during the Competitive Season, when we want to be as rested, fresh, and race-ready as possible.

Number of Sets, Repetitions, and Weight/Resistance Selection

The specific programs and routines presented in Chapters 2 and 3 will suggest the number of sets for each exercise and the number of repetitions to be completed within each set. Rest periods between sets will generally be brief—less than 30 seconds. To be even more time-efficient, many of our coached athletes limit their rest to 10 to 15 seconds between sets.

Another time-saving measure used by many of our coached athletes, and one we suggest, is a circuit-training approach. In other words, instead of doing three sets of an exercise and moving on to the next, athletes do one set of every exercise, then a second set, and finally a third set. This approach further shortens the rest time needed between sets because the muscles primarily used in one exercise can usually recover while you focus on the muscles needed for the next. The programs in this book are presented in a format to help facilitate this approach if you decide to try it.

For sets and repetitions that involve weights of some type, you should select the weight that allows you to complete the first set of that exercise within the suggested range of repetitions. For example, if the exercise indicates 8 to 12 repetitions, you should select a weight with which you can complete a maximum of 8 to 12 repetitions in the first set. Please note that if you can complete 8 to 12 repetitions in the first set, it's likely that you will only be able to complete some lesser number of repetitions in the second and third sets.

Once you find that you have become stronger and can now do more repetitions in the first set than the amount suggested, you should move up to a higher weight that puts you back into the suggested range on the first set. For example, if the exercise indicates 8 to 12 repetitions, once you can do more than 12 repetitions in the first set, you should move up in weight to bring you back into the 8-to-12-repetition range. Usually a 5 percent increase in weight will accomplish this.

Functional Strength- and Core-Training Equipment

As mentioned above, functional strength and core training has its own specific equipment. Following is a list of the suggested equipment to use in the exercises in Chapters 2 and 3:

1. BOSU Ball (acronym for "both sides utilized"): This is an inflated "half-ball" with a platform side and a half-dome side. This popular piece of equipment is primarily used to develop balance and stability on an uneven and/or unstable surface.
2. Dumbbells: These are the same traditional pieces of handheld exercise equipment familiar to most athletes. Dumbbells are available in various coatings from plastic to metal, and various weights from one pound to more than fifty pounds.
3. Foam Roller: These are usually 36 inches long with a 6-inch diameter, with varying densities.
4. Kettle Bells: These are handheld weights, but unlike dumbbells, the center of mass is extended beyond the hand. This facilitates ballistic and swinging movements. Like dumbbells, they are available in various weights.
5. Medicine Ball: This is a round, weighted ball often with a rubberized coating. It is available in various weights from one to twenty pounds.
6. Stability Ball/Swiss Ball: This round, inflated exercise ball is the most popular and widely used piece of core-training equipment. It is important that it be properly sized to fit your height. Following are our sizing suggestions based on an athlete's height:

   - 55cm diameter for 4 feet, 8 inches to 5 feet, 5 inches
   - 65cm diameter for 5 feet, 6 inches to 6 feet, 0 inches
   - 75cm diameter for 6 feet, 1 inch to 6 feet, 5 inches

7. Stretch Cords and Resistance Tubing: These are rubber or plastic cords, usually with handles, available in various resistances.

These items can be purchased at your local fitness/sports equipment store or online. Some helpful websites include:

performbetter.com
sportsauthority.com
dickssportinggoods.com

In Chapters 2 and 3 we will present several specific warm-up, stretching, and functional strength- and core-training programs. Each program is designed to be time-efficient and specific to your sport of choice. Not only will these programs build the kind of dynamic strength that will enable you to better transfer power through your body, but they will also help you to achieve better muscle balance and become more injury-proof. So, let's get started!

CHAPTER 2

Start Off on the Right Foot: Mind and Body Preparation

We have to do the best we can. This is our
sacred human responsibility.

—*Albert Einstein*

Upon waking in the morning, or after sitting at your desk for several hours, or after any other stationary activity you may have been doing prior to training, your body usually feels tight from decreased blood flow (and thus, decreased oxygen) to muscles, joints, and tendons.

Body Preparation and Warm-up

Before we begin any type of exercise, be it cardiovascular or strength training, we want to prepare our bodies. This often-overlooked part of training is especially important for endurance athletes who typically find that their muscles stiffen up during downtime. A proper warm-up is essential to a more-productive and safe cardio or strength session.

Before we begin to exercise, we need to raise our core body temperature and lubricate our joints and tendons. An efficient warm-up routine will do just that; in addition, it will increase the quality of the workout while reducing the risk of injury.

"Easy Eight"

Our coached athletes have had great success with a fast, efficient warm-up routine we like to call the "Easy Eight." These eight pre-movement exercises will help your body awaken from its sleeping or stationary state and prepare itself for the training ahead. The beauty of these exercises is the almost continuous flow from one body movement to the next.

While we should take short breaks between some of the exercises in our functional strength and core programs, such pauses should be avoided during our pre-exercise warm-up routine. We want to flow from one exercise to the next in a nice, fluid sequence, and, after having practiced it a few times, be able to complete this routine in less than five minutes. They are five minutes well spent, and will go a long way toward increasing the productivity of our workout, while decreasing the risk of injury. As with all the programs we design for time-crunched endurance athletes, the Easy Eight is short, sweet, and gets the job done.

While performing the Easy Eight exercises, focus on your breathing. You always want to start each exercise with an inhalation, and then exhale as you proceed through the movement. Be sure to breathe in through your nose and out through your mouth, while keeping your tongue on the roof of your mouth and your lips loose.

The Easy Eight Warm-up Routine

1. Pelvic Circles in Standing Position

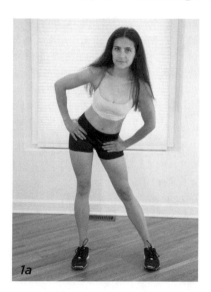 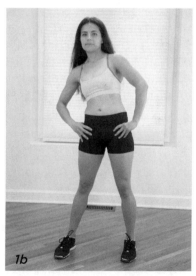

Start in a standing position with your feet at about the three o'clock and the nine o'clock positions, slightly beyond shoulder-width apart, with your hands on your hips. Begin with a deep breath in through your nose, exhale, and start by making a circular motion "around the clock" with your hips and pelvis. Go ten slow circles clockwise and then reverse with ten circles counterclockwise. This will help to increase blood flow and open up the hips and pelvis. (See photos 1a and 1b above.)

2. Chest Openers

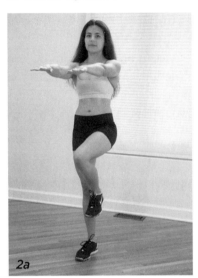
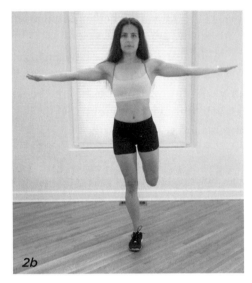

Start in a standing position with your feet slightly apart. Inhale, and begin by raising one leg off the ground with your hands at your sides. While exhaling, raise both arms straight out in front of you, with palms facing down, and then open your arms straight out to your sides as you rotate your palms toward the ceiling, simultaneously bringing your leg back so your quad is perpendicular to the floor. Bring arms back to front and repeat the movement five times before switching legs and repeating five more times. Be sure to maintain good posture throughout the movement by drawing your belly in and lifting your chest. (See photos 2a and 2b above.)

3. Three-Position Lunge (Front, 45°, side) with Opposite Arm Raise

Start in a standing position with your hands at your sides. Begin the movement by performing a forward lunge with your left leg while raising your

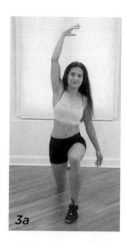
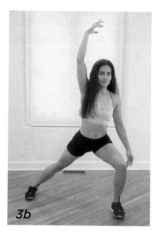
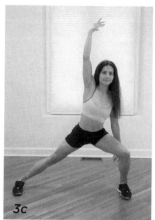

right arm, with palm up over your head. Press off your left foot, return arm to your side, and return to the start position. With your left leg, lunge again but at a forward angle of 45°, raising your right arm palm up over your head. Press off your left foot and return your arm back to your side as you return to the start position. Again with your left leg, lunge directly to the side while raising your right arm palm up over your head. Press off your left foot and return arm to your side as you return to the start position. Repeat this lunge pattern with your right leg and left arm. (See photos 3a, 3b, and 3c above.)

4. Forward Lunge with Elbow inside Knee

Start in a standing position and then lunge forward with your left leg while bringing your left elbow inside your left knee; place your right hand on the floor even with left foot. Hold that position for a 30-second count. Your knee should be over your ankle and your quadriceps should be at least parallel to the ground. Then take your left arm outside of your left knee and raise it straight up over your head, look toward the ceiling, and hold for a second. Then return your arm to the start position and repeat the arm raise four more times. Bring your left leg back even with your right foot and stand up. Repeat lunge with right leg and perform movement on that side. (See photos 4a and 4b on page 16.)

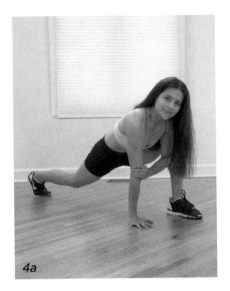

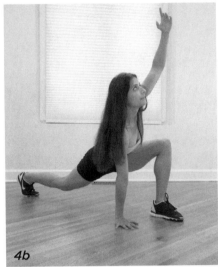

4a

4b

5. McKenzie Press-up

Start by lying flat on your stomach with your arms bent, palms near your shoulders and toes pointed. Begin the movement by inhaling, then exhale as you press up with your arms while keeping your hips on the floor and letting your stomach and back sag. Extend your arms fully without pulling your hips off the floor, if you can. Repeat this movement ten times. (See photos 5a and 5b below.)

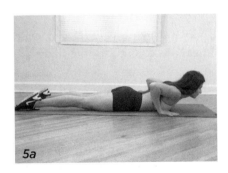

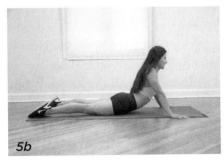

5a

5b

6. Kneeling Stretch

Starting from the up position of the McKenzie Press-up, sit back on your knees, keep your head down, extend your arms in front of you, and hold

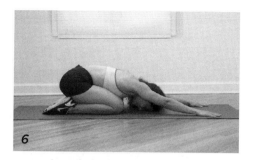

6

that stretch for 20 seconds. For an added stretch, allow your hips to drop slightly to one side and then repeat on the other side for a 20-second count. (See photo 6, left.)

7. Abs and Back Stretch over Stability Ball with Arms Overhead

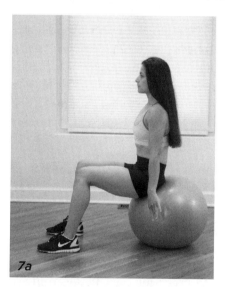

7a

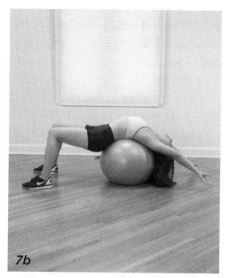

7b

Start by sitting on the stability ball and walk your feet out from it while your back follows the ball's contour as you lower it to the ball. Keep arms at your sides as you stretch your back and abs over the ball for a 30-second count. Then, extend your arms over your head and roll on the ball while keeping your head, neck, and back in contact with the ball. If you can, allow your hands to touch the floor behind you, hold, and then roll forward, letting your body follow the curve of the ball until you are almost sitting on the floor. At all times your head and back must be in contact with the ball. Roll forward and backward several times. (See photos 7a and 7b above.)

8. Torso Rotation over Stability Ball

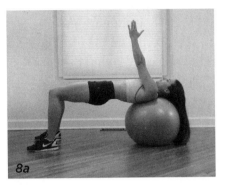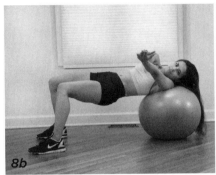

Start from the abdominal and back-stretch position in the previous exercise, but roll out on the ball so your head and neck are resting centered on the ball. Raise your arms straight up and bring your palms together. Roll your shoulders and torso to one side and bring your arms with you. Roll from side to side with arms and hips extended, feet apart. Repeat this ten times. (See photos 8a and 8b above.)

There you have it. In only about five minutes, the Easy Eight has prepared your body for a productive workout, while reducing the risk of injury. The Easy Eight warm-up routine can be very helpful before any training session, but especially so for training sessions done in the morning and after any other situations when you have been immobile for several hours, like sitting at your desk.

But we're not done yet. In addition to preparing their bodies to train, successful athletes must also prepare their minds. We don't want to stumble into our training while still stressed out from work or preoccupied with something else. To get the most from our training time, we want to be mentally relaxed and properly focused on having a productive and safe training session.

The following are some of our favorite and most effective relaxation, breathing, and visualization exercises that we have successfully used with our coached athletes. Work with these exercises to center your mind and hone your focus in order to maximize your training results.

Breathing and Relaxation Exercises

We are often amazed at the number of times in a day when we find ourselves telling our coached athletes, "Don't hold your breath!" or "Breathe!," or asking, "Are you holding your breath?" If you hold your breath and try to perform an exercise of any type—from strength training to swimming—it makes the task much more difficult, if not impossible.

One of our favorite Olympic events is the biathlon—cross-country skiing at 10km or 20km with two or four stops to fire a gun at a very small target. Miss the target, and you get a 1-minute penalty added to your skiing time, or you have to do an extra 150-meter loop, depending on the event distance. The difficulty of this sport is the jarring contrast between skiing very fast and stopping on a dime to shoot at a very small target with a rifle and (hopefully) very steady hands. Besides the obvious, the most difficult aspect is controlling your breathing when it comes time to shoot. To shoot accurately, most competitors utilize a technique of taking several deep breaths and then shooting at the end of the last exhalation. To us, the biathlete's task is the perfect example of how breathing controls one's performance.

How often have you heard a triathlete, runner, or open-water swimmer say that they hyperventilated at the start of a race? It's pretty common, but it doesn't have to be. If we can learn to control our breathing, we can avoid those situations.

Learning to breathe properly and effectively provides many health benefits, from relaxation and stress reduction to energizing and healing. We can learn to breathe much deeper to bring about positive change in our training and performance. Take note of your breathing right now. Are you breathing through your mouth with a short chest breath? Or are you exhaling through your mouth and inhaling through your nose? If you aren't doing the latter, you should be, but this definitely takes some practice and retraining of the mind and body.

There are various techniques of breathing, from yoga breathing (pranayama) to rhythmic and belly breathing. All of these techniques have benefits and can be used by most endurance athletes either to reduce stress and/or to bring increased blood flow to tired and fatigued muscles, and possibly to heal injuries.

Deep Belly Breathing

A breathing technique that we prefer to use before training and racing is deep belly breathing. You start by lying on the floor with one hand on your solar plexus and the other at or below your belly button. With the tip of your tongue lightly touching behind your upper front teeth, exhale through your mouth with relaxed lips before you begin an inhalation through your nose, attempting to bring the breath all the way to your lower abdomen. Then hold your breath for a count of 3 seconds before you exhale through your mouth for at least 6 to 10 seconds. Try to exhale for twice as long as your inhalation at a minimum. You can also do this in a sitting position while maintaining very good posture.

If you start doing this type of breathing a couple times per day, with five to six belly breaths each time, you will become very comfortable with the technique and be able to work its benefits into many situations. Use it to reduce pre-race nervousness, or any other time you can benefit from calming and relaxing your mind and body.

Visualization Technique: "Been There, Done That"

Mental preparation started for coauthor Don way back in high-school cross-country. He had most of his races then at the same course, at Warinanco Park in Elizabeth, New Jersey. He raced the course so many times that he knew every inch of it. The 2.5 miles wound through the park and then finished on the track in a stadium for the last quarter-mile.

In the days and hours leading up to a race, Don would visualize the entire race and how he expected it to unfold. He was a "kicker," which, as some of you know, means that he had a pretty good sprint, so he would try to run just behind the leader and stay as relaxed as possible for almost the entire race. Then, as the racers entered the track for the last quarter-mile, Don would try to drop it into another gear and blow past the leader, getting over the finish line first. Sometimes it worked, sometimes it didn't, but Don always went into the race with a very clear visualization of how it would unfold chronologically.

Don would visualize the mass start across a long field and then the runners all crowding into a path around the park. Don usually knew the kids

AN IRONFIT MOMENT

Foam Roller—Self-Massage and Myofascial Release

The foam roller can be used for self-massage and myofascial release. It is a great way to prepare yourself for a workout, as well as help you to recover from a workout. Originally, foam-roller use started as a way to apply pressure to a specific area of sensitivity, a knot, or even a trigger point. It has since progressed, and athletes now use it as a way to do self-massage with longer sweeping motions along various muscles like your quadriceps, hamstrings, calves, glutes, and back, both before and after workouts. For those athletes who are injury-prone or slow to recover, we recommend you pick up a foam roller and incorporate it into your warm-up or cooldown routine. They come in various densities, so choose the one that you can tolerate, and be sure to study the instructions and diagrams of various techniques of using the foam roller. If your foam roller does not come with such material, you can find instructions in our *Mastering the Marathon* book and other online sources.

from the other schools, so he would visualize who he would be running with and how the pack would likely dwindle as the race went on. Don would visualize his rivals putting in a surge at certain points to try to drop him, and he would visualize himself hanging with them while staying as relaxed as he could.

Visualization was a very powerful tool for Don, and although he didn't win them all, he won his share, and his preparation seemed to keep him competitive and in the game. Don felt confident, relaxed, and focused before and during the race because he always had that *been there, done that* feeling.

Don realized over the years that this type of mental preparation was not for race days only. He found that he benefited from preparing for all of his training in this same way. In no place is this truer than in strength training. Instead of blindly stumbling into our exercises half focused, we will gain much greater benefit if we visualize the entire workout in advance. Let's get dialed in mentally to each exercise in terms of what it focuses on and what we will gain from it. This approach will greatly enhance the benefits of our strength-training sessions. We want to approach them with that "been there, done that" mind-set. It's almost as if we have already completed the session before we start, because we have already executed it flawlessly in our minds.

So in addition to using the above warm-up routine to prepare your body for each strength-training session, also consider using the belly breathing technique and the "been there, done that" mental approach in order to prepare your mind, as well. These three approaches will work together to keep our strength and core training efficient and productive.

In addition to body preparation and warm-up, we also suggest you work on stretching—but after a long cardio workout or a strength-training session, not before. You might want to focus on your problem areas or those areas that are normally tight for you. We present various stretching routines in our books *Be Iron Fit, 2nd Edition* and *Mastering the Marathon*. If you have the time, you will want to supplement your strength training with some post-exercise stretching.

Now that we have discussed our suggested warm-up routine, breathing and relaxation exercises, and visualization technique, we will advance to Chapter 3 and our nine sport-specific functional strength and core programs.

The Optimal Strength- and Core-Training Program for You

The harder the conflict,
the more glorious the triumph.

—*Thomas Paine*

In the pages that follow in this chapter, you will find eleven highly efficient functional strength and core programs.

First we will introduce the "Fink Five," the five key exercises to be included at the start of each sport-specific program. Next we will present the nine sport-specific programs. Finally, we will describe a special program to be used in situations when, due to travel or other reasons, the athlete does not have the proper equipment or facilities to do his or her sport-specific program.

Please remember that each of the nine sport-specific routines begins with the Fink Five and then builds additional exercises on top of the Five. In the Off-Season Phase, which focuses on strength, you will be performing five specific exercises after the Fink Five, for a total of ten exercises. In the Preseason Phase, which focuses on power, and the Competitive-Season Phase, which focuses on maintenance, you will perform only three exercises after the Fink Five, for a total of eight exercises.

Most athletes can complete the Fink Five and Off-Season Phase exercises together in less than 25 minutes, and they can complete the Fink Five and Preseason or Competitive-Season exercises in less than 20 minutes. If you start with the Easy Eight warm-up routine from Chapter 2, a complete strength warm-up and workout can be finished in less than 30 minutes and 25 minutes, respectively. This tight time requirement fits in well with most good sport-specific training programs (i.e., run, bike, swim, etc.) because the strength-program training time gets shorter as the primary sports-training time grows.

In addition to each program being presented in three phases—Off-Season, Preseason, and Competitive-Season—it is also presented in three levels of progression. Once the Basic level of each exercise is mastered, the athlete may then progress to the Intermediate level. Once the Intermediate level is mastered, the athlete will graduate to the Advanced level.

And now, here they are: the Fink Five, the nine sport-specific functional strength- and core-training programs, and a special travel program.

Functional Strength and Core Programs:

1. The Fink Five, page 24
2. Long-Course Triathlete (Half-Iron to Ultra Distance), page 32
3. Short-Course Triathlete (Sprint to Olympic Distance), page 47
4. Runners–Road Racer (5K to Full Marathon), page 59
5. Runners–Ultra Distance (50K to 100 miles), page 70
6. Distance Cyclist, page 81
7. Swimmers—Distance and Open-Water, page 91
8. Cross-Country Skier, page 101
9. Duathlete, page 112
10. Adventure Racer, page 122
11. Special Travel Program, page 132

The Fink Five

The Fink Five will always be our first five exercises of each functional strength-training session throughout the year.

1. Squats with Dumbbells
2. Back Lunge with Overhead Reach Using Dumbbell
3. Transverse Lunge with Stretch Cord or Cable Row
4. Straight-Leg or Bent-Knee Push-up
5. Planks with Rollout on Knees and Forearms on Stability Ball

1. Squats with Dumbbells

Purpose: To strengthen glutes, hamstrings, quads, and core.

Basic: Squats with Dumbbells—Stability Ball against the Wall

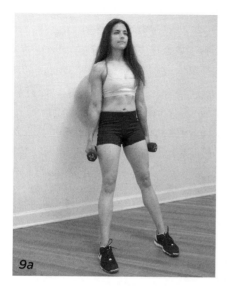

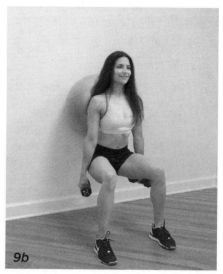

9a

9b

Start in a standing position with the stability ball against the wall, centered at your lower back. Your feet are about shoulder-width apart and you have a dumbbell in each hand at your sides. Begin by inhaling and shifting your hips back and bending your knees into a squat position, bringing your quadriceps parallel to the floor. Then, exhale as you extend your legs back to the standing position. (See photos 9a and 9b above.)

Intermediate: Squats with Dumbbells on BOSU

Same as the Basic except you are standing on BOSU, without your back touching a stability ball. Press hips back and avoid arching your back. (See photo 9c, right.)

Advanced: One-Leg Squat with Dumbbells

Start in a standing position not on the BOSU, holding a dumbbell in

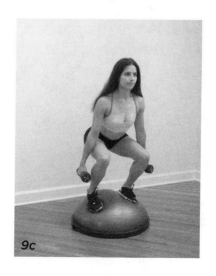

9c

25

each hand. Raise one leg off the ground, and then extend it behind you as you perform a squat on the other leg. Hold, and then return to the start position without placing the foot on the ground. Repeat for the desired number of repetitions. Switch legs and perform the same number of repetitions on the other leg.

Sets/Reps: Off-Season—three sets of 8 to 12 reps / Preseason— three sets of 12 to 15 reps / Competitive Season—three sets of 20 reps / Advanced: Off-Season—three sets of 8 to 12 reps, each leg / Preseason—three sets of 10 to 12 reps, each leg / Competitive Season—three sets of 15 reps, each leg

2. Back Lunge with Overhead Reach Using Dumbbell

Purpose: To strengthen glutes, hamstrings, quads, obliques, core, and balance.

Basic: Back Lunge with Overhead Reach Using Dumbbell

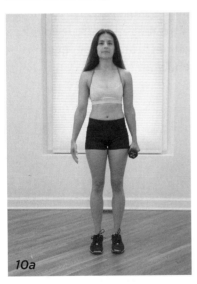
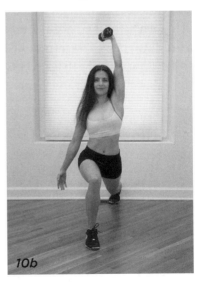

10a

10b

Start in a standing position with a light dumbbell in one hand. Take a step back with the same side leg as the hand with the dumbbell. As you step back into a lunge position, raise your arm to the side with a slight bend, palm

26

facing up in an arching motion over your head. Then, extend your hips, glutes, and quads to return to the start position and simultaneously return your arm to your side. Repeat repetitions on that leg/arm and before switching to the other leg/arm. (See photos 10a and 10b, left.)

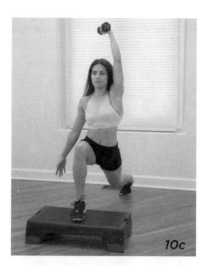

Intermediate: Back Lunge off Step with Overhead Reach Using Dumbbell

Same as the Basic, except start by standing on a step. (See photo 10c, right.)

10c

Advanced: Back Lunge off BOSU with Overhead Reach Using Dumbbell

Same as Intermediate, except start by standing on a BOSU with one foot more centered on the BOSU and the other just touching lightly next to it.

Sets/Reps: Off-Season—three sets of 8 to 12 reps each leg / Preseason—three sets of 10 to 12 reps, each leg / Competitive Season—three sets of 15 reps, each leg

3. Transverse Lunge with Stretch Cord or Cable Row

Purpose: To strengthen glutes, hamstrings, quads, shoulders, back, core, and balance.

Basic: Transverse Lunge with Stretch Cord or Cable Row

Start in a standing position facing forward with the stretch cord or cable in your right hand and arm extended straight, about shoulder height. The stretch cord/band should have sufficient tension on it. Perform a transverse lunge (lunge back at 45° angle) by rotating your entire body to the right, keeping your left foot planted. Simultaneously, pull the cord/band toward your shoulder by bending your elbow back but keeping your arm parallel to

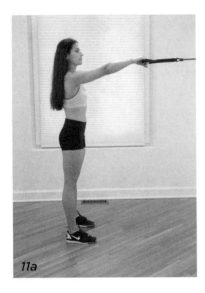
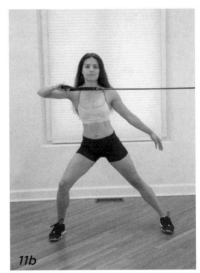

the floor with a 1-second hold. Then, return to the start position and repeat for the desired number of repetitions with that arm before switching to the other arm. (See photos 11a and 11b above.)

Intermediate: Transverse Lunge onto Step with Stretch Cord or Cable Row

Same as the Basic, except the lunging leg lands on a step.

Advanced: Transverse Lunge onto BOSU with Stretch Cord or Cable Row

Same as the Basic, except the lunging leg lands on a BOSU.

Sets/Reps: Off-Season—three sets of 8 to 12 reps each leg / Preseason—three sets of 10 to 12 reps, each leg / Competitive Season—three sets of 15 reps, each leg

4. Straight-Leg or Bent-Knee Push-up

Purpose: To strengthen chest, shoulders, triceps, abs, and core.

Basic: Straight-Leg or Bent-Knee Push-up

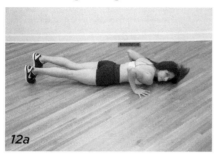

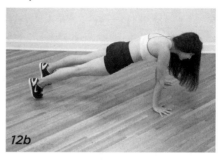

Start by lying facedown on the floor with your arms bent and hands to the outside of your shoulders. Raise your torso, head, and legs off the floor by extending your arms straight into a plank position to get to the start position. While holding a straight line from your ankles to your shoulders, and keeping your head in alignment with your spine, lower your chest toward the floor and hold for 1 second before pushing your body back into the straight-line position. Breathe in on the way down and exhale on the exertion. Repeat for the desired number of repetitions. (See photos 12a and 12b above.)

Intermediate: Straight-Leg or Bent-Knee Traveling Push-up

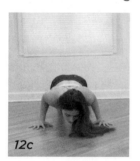

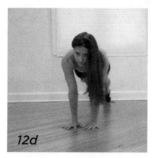

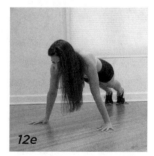

Same as the Basic, except after you perform one push-up and return to the start position (arms extended), one at a time, move one hand 12 inches inward or outward and the other hand 12 inches similarly in or out. Perform another push-up and repeat the traveling motion back toward the other direction (outward or inward). You can also do this by traveling across a step or BOSU. (See photos 12c, 12d, and 12e above.)

Advanced: Straight-Leg Push-up with One Leg Raised

Same as the Basic, except in the starting position raise one leg so it is parallel to the ground but not touching; perform half the number of repetitions on one leg, and then raise the other leg and perform the remaining number of repetitions.

Sets/Reps: Off-Season—three sets of 8 to 12 reps / Preseason—three sets of 10 to 12 reps / Competitive Season—three sets of 15 to 20 reps

5. Planks with Rollout on Knees and Forearms on Stability Ball

Purpose: To strengthen shoulders, back, abdominals, and core.

Basic: Planks with Rollout on Knees and Forearms on Stability Ball

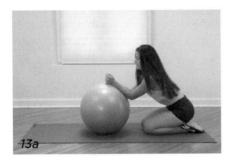 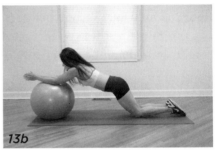

Start by kneeling in front of a stability ball with your forearms and hands together on the front part of the ball. Raise your torso in a straight line and slowly roll the ball out from your body with your forearms until you feel your abdominals engaging, without arching your back. Hold for 3 to 5 seconds and then return to the start position. (See photos 13a and 13b above.)

Intermediate: Planks on Toes and Forearms on Stability Ball

Same as the Basic, except start on your toes (not on your knees), and roll the ball out so that your legs are straight and your forearms are on the stability ball, with your body in a straight line from your shoulders to your ankles. Hold this position for 30 to 60 seconds. Then, return to the start position.

Advanced: Planks on Toes with One Leg Raised

Same as the Intermediate, except raise one leg and hold for 15 to 60 seconds and then repeat with the other leg raised.

Sets/Reps: Off-Season—three sets of 8 to 12 reps / Preseason—three sets of 10 to 12 reps / Competitive Season—three sets of 15 reps / Intermediate and Advanced: Off-Season—three sets of 15 to 30 seconds / Preseason—three sets of 30 to 45 seconds / Competitive Season—three sets of 30 to 60 seconds

Long-Course Triathlete Program

(Half-Iron to Ultra Distance Triathlons)

This program includes the following exercises:

Off-Season	Preseason	Competitive Season
Fink Five	Fink Five	Fink Five
1. Ax Chop on BOSU	1. Lateral Lunge	1. Pullovers on Stability Ball
2. Chest Flys	2. One-Leg Press/	2. Superman on BOSU
3. Side Lunge with	Hop	3. Overhead Raises
Front Raise	3. Get-ups	
4. Rear Delt Flys		
5. Ab Triangles		

First Phase: Off-Season of Long-Course Triathlete Program

In the Off-Season, the Long-Course Triathlete Program starts with the Fink Five and then goes right into the following five exercises, which most practiced athletes can complete in less than 12 minutes. If an athlete starts with the Easy Eight warm-up routine (5 minutes), then completes the Fink Five (12 minutes), and then finishes up with the following five exercises (12 minutes), he or she can complete the entire Off-Season Program in under 30 minutes.

1. Squat with Ax Chop on BOSU

Purpose: To strengthen hamstrings, quads, glutes, abdominals, arms, shoulders, back, and core.

Basic: Squat with Ax Chop on BOSU Using Medicine Ball

Start by standing on top of the BOSU and holding a medicine ball at shoulder height to one side, with arms bent. As you are performing a squat, and at the same pace as the squat, lower the medicine ball to the opposite side across your body in a chopping motion until you complete the squat. Return to the

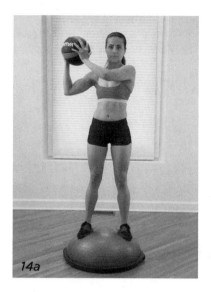
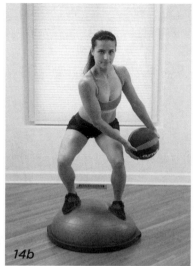

start position, extending the legs while reversing the chopping motion, and then repeat on the same side before switching to the other side. (See photos 14a and 14b above.)

Intermediate: Squat with Ax Chop on BOSU Using Kettle Bell

Same as the Basic, except use a kettle bell to perform the exercise.

Advanced: Side Lunge with Ax Chop on BOSU Using Kettle Bell

Start by standing on top of the BOSU and holding a kettle bell at shoulder height to one side, with arms bent. As you are performing a side lunge, swing the kettle bell to the opposite side across your body in a chopping motion to the outside of your lunging leg until you complete the lunge. Return to the start position and bring the kettle bell back to the opposite shoulder by reversing the chopping motion. Repeat on the opposite side.

Sets/Reps: Off-Season—three sets of 8 to 12 reps on each side

2. Chest Flys with Stretch Cords in Lunge Position

Purpose: To strengthen pectorals, shoulders, glutes, hamstrings, abdominals, core, and balance.

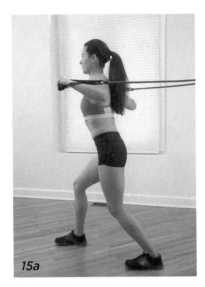
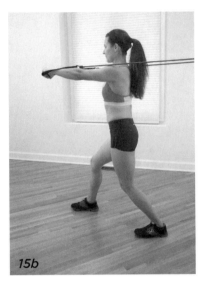

15a 15b

Basic: Chest Flys with Stretch Cords in Lunge Position

Start in a standing position holding the ends of the stretch cord in both hands, facing away from the door/wall with your legs in a lunge position. Extend your slightly bent arms out to the sides about chest level. Inhale, then exhale as you squeeze your chest and bring your arms together in front with palms facing down, hold, then return to the start position while keeping your arms extended from your sides. (See photos 15a and 15b above.)

Intermediate: Chest Flys with Stretch Cords—Standing on One Leg

Same as the Basic, except start by standing on one leg. Perform the movement with one leg raised for half of the repetitions, and then repeat with the other leg raised for the other half of the repetitions.

Advanced: Alternating Arm/Chest Flys with Stretch Cords—Standing on One Leg

Same as the Intermediate, except with leg raised, perform the movement with alternating arms. Start with both arms extended in front of you and then perform a fly with only one arm. Perform half of the repetitions on one leg and then switch legs and perform the remaining repetitions.

Sets/Reps: Off-Season—three sets of 8 to 12 reps

3. Side Lunge with Front Raise

Purpose: To strengthen glutes, hamstrings, quads, ab/adductors, shoulders, and core.

Basic: Side Lunge with Front Raise

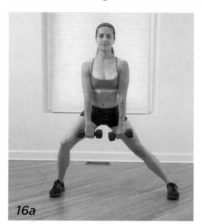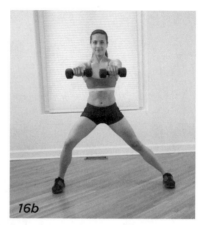

16a 16b

Start in a standing position with a dumbbell in each hand at your sides. Perform a side lunge, keeping your hips back and lunging leg bent while your other leg stays straight. From that position, raise your arms with dumbbells out straight to shoulder height, hold, and then simultaneously bring your arms back to your sides while extending your hips, glutes, and quads back to the start position. Perform half of the repetitions on one leg and then switch and perform half of the repetitions on the other leg. (See photos 16a and 16b above.)

Intermediate: Side Lunge onto Step with Front Raise

Same as the Basic, except side-lunge onto a step.

Advanced: Side Lunge onto BOSU with One-Arm Front Raise

Same as the Intermediate, except side-lunge onto a BOSU so your foot strikes the center of it, and raise the same side arm. Then, repeat with other leg and arm.

Sets/Reps: Off-Season—three sets of 8 to 12 reps / Advanced—three sets of 8 to 12 reps, each side

4. Rear Deltoid Flys in a Stork Position

Purpose: To strengthen deltoids, rhomboids, hamstrings, quads, core, and balance.

Basic: Rear Deltoid Flys in Stork Position

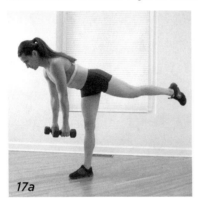 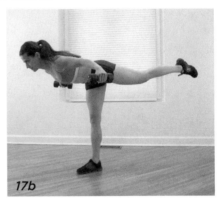

17a   17b

Start in a standing position with a dumbbell in each hand. Raise one leg straight behind you and balance on the other leg in a stork position, letting your arms hang straight down. Depress your shoulder blades toward your spine and raise the dumbbells with slightly bent arms out to the sides, but not higher than shoulder height. Hold for a 2-second count and then return arms back to the start position and repeat. Keep hands soft as you squeeze your shoulder blades together to elevate the weights. Perform half the repetitions on one leg and then switch and perform half the repetitions on the other leg. (See photos 17a and 17b above.)

Intermediate: Rear Deltoid Flys in Stork Position, Alternating Arms

Same as the Basic, except perform this exercise by raising one arm at a time and alternating arms. Perform half of the repetitions on one leg and then switch and perform half of the repetitions on the other leg.

Advanced: Rear Deltoid Flys with One-Leg Squat in Stork Position

Same as the Basic, except start this exercise from the stork position and begin with a one-leg squat. Then, as you extend from the squat, simultaneously raise the weights as you return to the start position. Perform half of the repetitions on one leg and then switch and perform half of the repetitions on the other leg.

Sets/Reps: Off-Season—three sets of 8 to 12 reps

5. Abs—Open-and-Close Triangles

Purpose: To strengthen overall core and abdominals.

Basic: Abs—Open-and-Close Triangles

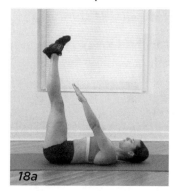 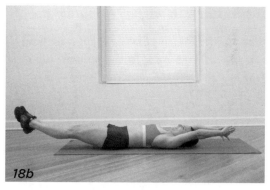

Start by lying on the floor on your back with legs extended straight, so they are perpendicular to the floor, and your arms extended toward your knees. Your legs, torso, and arms should almost form a right triangle. Simultaneously, lower your legs together toward the floor and your arms straight over your head from your shoulders. Hold your position when you are straight but not quite touching the ground, and then return to the start position and repeat. (See photos 18a and 18b above.)

Intermediate: Abs—Stability Ball Pass from Hands to Feet

Same as the Basic, except you start with a stability ball in your hands as you lower your arms overhead and your legs toward the floor. Then, simultaneously, raise your arms and legs together and pass the stability ball from your hands to between your feet and repeat the movement. Continue passing the ball from your hands to your feet at each return to starting point and make the movement continuous. (See photos 18c and 18d, next page.)

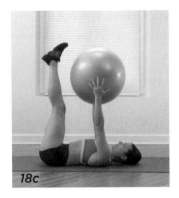
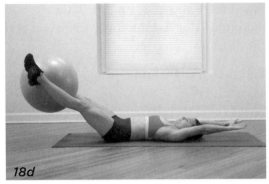

Advanced: Stability Ball Pass from Hands to Feet with Raised Torso

Same as the Intermediate, except raise your torso off the floor every time you raise your arms back to the straight position, with or without the stability ball.

Sets/Reps: Off-Season—three sets of 8 to 12 reps

Second Phase: Preseason of Long-Course Triathlete Program (reps increase to 10–15 range)

Once we are about eight to twelve weeks away from our first major race of the year, we will transition into the Preseason Phase of the Long-Course Triathlete Program. This phase starts with the Fink Five and then goes right into the following three exercises, which most practiced athletes can complete in about 7.5 minutes. If an athlete starts with the Easy Eight warm-up routine (5 minutes), then completes the Fink Five (12 minutes), and then finishes up with the following three Preseason Exercises (7.5 minutes), he or she can complete the entire Preseason Program in under 25 minutes.

1. Lateral Lunge/Squat across BOSU

Purpose: To strengthen glutes, hamstrings, quads, ankles, core, balance, and power.

Basic: Lateral Lunge/Squat across BOSU

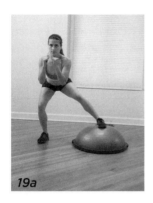
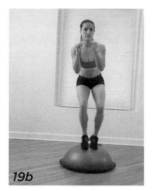
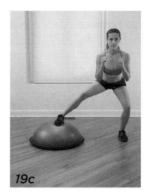

19a   19b   19c

Start by standing on the BOSU. Then, take one leg and lunge to the side into a deep squat, keeping your other foot on the BOSU. Then quickly jump your off foot onto the BOSU and lunge with the other leg to the opposite side. Repeat side to side quickly while maintaining good form. (see photos 19a, 19b, and 19c above.)

Intermediate: Lateral Lunge/Squat across BOSU with Medicine Ball Reach

Start by standing on the BOSU with a medicine ball at chest height, with bent arms. Take one leg and lunge to the side into a deep squat, keeping your other foot on the BOSU while simultaneously extending the medicine ball straight out in front of you. Bring the medicine ball back to your chest and then quickly jump your off foot onto the BOSU; then, lunge with the other leg to the opposite side while reaching out front again with the medicine ball. Repeat side to side quickly while maintaining good form.

Advanced: Lateral Lunge/Squat across BOSU with 180° Turn

Start by standing on the BOSU. Take one leg and lunge to the side into a deep squat, keeping the other foot on the BOSU. Then, quickly jump straight up with both legs and simultaneously make a 180° turn so you face the opposite direction, landing with the opposite foot on the BOSU and the other foot on the ground. Jump across the BOSU and repeat 180° turn on that side. Repeat side to side quickly with the 180° turn while maintaining good form. (See photos 19d, 19e, and 19f, next page.)

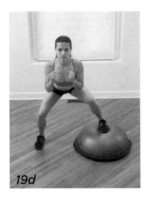
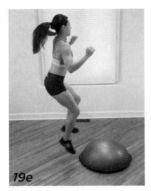
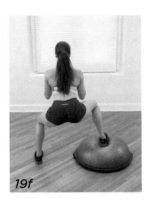

19d   19e   19f

Sets/Reps: Preseason—three sets of 10 to 12 reps

2. One-Leg Press to Hop (with or without dumbbells)

Purpose: To strengthen glutes, hamstrings, quads, ankles, core, and balance, and to develop power.

Basic: One-Leg Press with Foot on Step (with or without dumbbells)

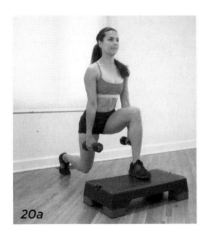
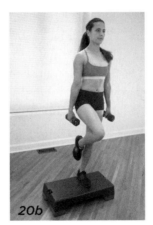

20a   20b

Start by standing in a lunge position with one foot on the step and the other foot behind, with knee bent almost to the floor. Perform a one-leg press with the leg on the step, and rise to a standing position while bringing the opposite leg up with raised knee. Return to the start position and repeat on that leg, and then switch to the other leg. (See photos 20a and 20b above.)

Intermediate: One-Leg Press to Hop with Foot on Step (with or without dumbbells)

Same as the Basic, except after you complete the press, hop on the same leg while keeping the opposite leg raised in a chair pose. Return to the start position and repeat on the same leg before switching to the opposite leg for the remaining repetitions. (See photo 20c, right.)

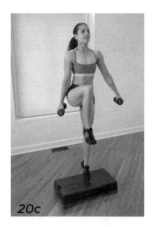

20c

Advanced: One-Leg Press to Hop with Foot on BOSU (with or without dumbbells)

Same as the Intermediate, except start with one foot on the BOSU; then, after you complete the press, hop on that same leg while raising the opposite knee in a chair pose. Repeat on the same leg before switching to the opposite leg.

Sets/Reps: Preseason—three sets of 10 to 12 reps, each leg

3. Get-ups off BOSU with Arms at Your Sides

Purpose: To strengthen core and abdominals, glutes, quads, core, and hamstrings

Basic: Get-ups off the BOSU with Arms at Your Sides

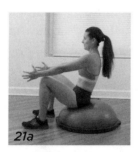
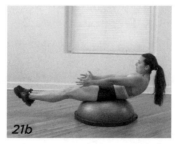
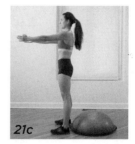

21a   21b   21c

Start by sitting on the BOSU, with arms at your sides and bent knees. Extend your torso back so you are completely parallel to the floor and legs are raised off the floor. Then, raise torso and simultaneously put your feet on the floor and stand straight up. Then, return to the start position and repeat. (See photos 21a, 21b, and 21c above.)

Intermediate: Get-ups off BOSU with Arms Raised

Same as the Basic, except with both arms extended over your head for the entire exercise. Raise your torso and simultaneously bring your feet to the floor and stand up, keeping arms extended over your head.

Advanced: Get-ups off Floor with Medicine Ball Overhead

Same as the Intermediate, except start by lying on the floor instead of the BOSU, with knees bent and holding a medicine ball over your head. As you begin to "get up," bring the ball down from over your head to in front of your chest.

Sets/Reps: Preseason—three sets of 10 to 12 reps

Third Phase: Competitive Season of Long-Course Triathlete Program (reps increase to 15–20 range)

Once we have completed our first major race of the year, we will transition into the Competitive-Season Phase of the Long-Course Triathlete Program. This phase starts with the Fink Five and then goes right into the following three exercises, which most practiced athletes can complete in about 5 minutes. If an athlete starts with the Easy Eight warm-up routine (5 minutes), then completes the Fink Five (12 minutes), and then finishes up with the following three Competitive-Season Exercises (7.5 minutes), he or she can complete the entire Competitive-Season Program in less than 25 minutes. Additional Note: As part of a proper pre-race taper, it is our general suggestion not to perform strength training during the week immediately preceding a major race.

1. Pullovers with Hip Extension on Stability Ball Using Medicine Ball

Purpose: To strengthen lats, pectorals, glutes, hamstrings, and core.

Basic: Pullovers with Hip Extension on Stability Ball Using Medicine Ball

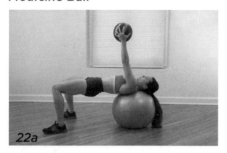
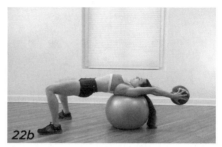

Start by lying on the stability ball with your back, neck, and head resting on top of the ball and your hips extended and knees bent, keeping quadriceps parallel to the floor. Raise the medicine ball with arms straight above your chest, inhale, and keep hips and knees in a straight line as you extend the medicine ball over your head, bringing your arms as close to parallel to the floor as possible. Hold that position for 1 second, and then while exhaling, raise the ball back to the start position and repeat. (See photos 22a and 22b above.)

Intermediate: Pullovers on Stability Ball with Dumbbells

Same as the Basic, except that you use a dumbbell in each hand and perform the same movement with elbows slightly bent.

Advanced: Pullovers on Stability Ball with Medicine Ball and One Leg Raised

Same as the Basic, except you perform the exercise with one leg raised.

Sets/Reps: Competitive Season—three sets of 12 to 15 reps

2. Superman on BOSU

Purpose: To strengthen back, shoulders, glutes, hamstrings, abdominals, and core.

Basic: Superman on BOSU

Start by lying facedown with your hips centered on the BOSU, your legs straight and hip-width apart, and your palms facing up. Extend your shoulder

43

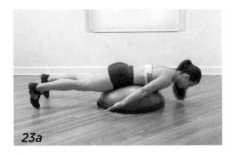
23a

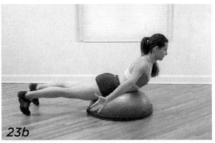
23b

blades back and down toward your spine. Inhale to prepare for the movement, and then exhale as you extend your lower back, squeezing your glutes as you extend your torso up while rotating your thumbs toward the ceiling. Hold for 1 second in that position before returning to the start position. (See photos 23a and 23b above.)

Intermediate: Superman on BOSU with Arms Overhead

Same as the Basic, except raise your arms over your head and perform the movement without rotating your thumbs toward the ceiling. (See photo 23c, right.)

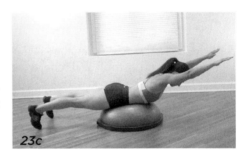
23c

Advanced: Swimming on BOSU

Start by lying facedown, balanced on your midsection over the BOSU, with legs extended and arms overhead. Raise your arms and legs off the floor, find your balance, and then perform a swimming-type movement by fluttering your arms and legs for about 30 to 60 seconds. (See photo 23d above.)

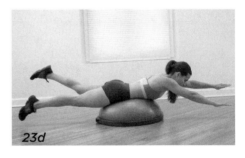
23d

Sets/Reps: Competitive Season—three sets of 12 to 15 reps
Advanced: Sets/Reps: Competitive Season—three sets of 30 to 60 seconds

3. Overhead Raises with Stretch Cords or Bands

Purpose: To strengthen shoulders, back, lats, abdominals, and core.

Basic: Overhead Raises with Stretch Cords or Bands

Start by holding one end of a stretch cord in both hands and place your foot on the other end of the stretch cord on the floor to hold it in place. Give yourself enough slack so you can extend the stretch cord directly over your head, keeping your arms straight. While keeping your arms straight, raise the stretch cord directly above your shoulders and head; then, lower to start position and repeat.

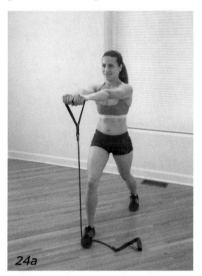
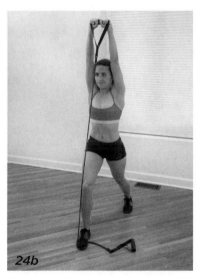

24a

24b

Intermediate: Overhead Raises with Stretch Cords or Bands in Lunge Position

Same as the Basic, except stagger your feet in a lunge position while raising the stretch cord directly over your head. Split the repetitions between each leg. (See photos 24a and 24b above.)

Advanced: Squat with Overhead Raises Using Kettle Bell

Start by standing with feet shoulder-width apart, holding one kettle bell with both hands. Begin by squatting back and bringing the kettle bell through

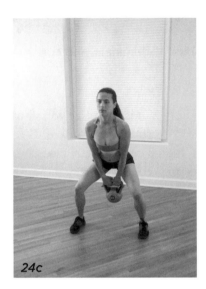
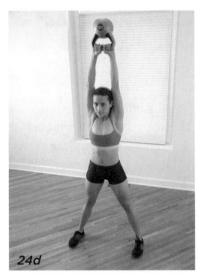

your legs. Then, while extending out of the squat and returning to a standing position, simultaneously swing the kettle bell straight out in front and above your head while keeping your arms straight. Then, slowly lower the kettle bell and return to the start position. (See photos 24c and 24d above.)

Sets/Reps: Competitive Season—three sets of 12 to 15 reps

Short-Course Triathlete Program

(Sprint to Olympic Distance Triathlons)

This program includes the following exercises:

Off-Season	Preseason	Competitive Season
Fink Five	Fink Five	Fink Five
1. Ax Chop on BOSU	1. Lateral Lunge	1. Rear Delt Flys
2. Chest Press	2. One-Leg Press/	2. Superman on BOSU
3. Jump Squats	Hop	3. Overhead Raises
4. Side Lunge with	3. Get-ups	
Front Raise		
5. Obliques		

First Phase: Off-Season of Short-Course Triathlete Program

In the Off-Season, the Short-Course Triathlete Program starts with the Fink Five and then goes right into the following five exercises, which most practiced athletes can complete in 12 minutes. If an athlete starts with the Easy Eight warm-up routine (5 minutes), then completes the Fink Five (12 minutes), and then finishes up with the following five exercises (12 minutes), he or she can complete the entire Off-Season Program in less than 30 minutes.

1. Squat with Ax Chop on BOSU

Purpose: To strengthen hamstrings, quads, glutes, abdominals, arms, shoulders, core, and back.

Basic: Squat with Ax Chop on BOSU Using Medicine Ball

Start by standing on top of the BOSU and holding a medicine ball at shoulder height to one side, with arms bent. As you are performing a squat, and at the same pace as the squat, lower the medicine ball to the opposite side across your body in a chopping motion until you complete the squat. Return to the start position, extending the legs while reversing the chopping motion, and then repeat on the same side before switching to the other side. (See page 33.)

Intermediate: Squat with Ax Chop on BOSU Using Kettle Bell

Same as the Basic, except use a kettle bell to perform the exercise.

Advanced: Side Lunge with Ax Chop on BOSU Using Kettle Bell

Start by standing on top of the BOSU and holding a kettle bell at shoulder height to one side, with arms bent. As you are performing a side lunge, swing the kettle bell to the opposite side across your body in a chopping motion to the outside of your lunging leg until you complete the lunge. Return to the start position and bring the kettle bell back to the opposite shoulder by reversing the chopping motion. Repeat on the opposite side.

Sets/Reps: Off-Season—three sets of 8 to 12 reps on each side

2. Chest Press over Stability Ball with Hip Extension

Purpose: To strengthen pectorals, deltoids, triceps, glutes, hamstrings, abdominals, and balance.

Basic: Chest Press over Stability Ball with Hip Extension

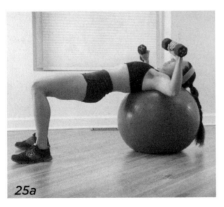
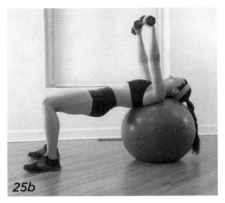

25a

25b

Start by lying with your head and neck centered on top of the stability ball, with your hips extended and knees bent to create a straight line from your knees to your shoulders. With arms bent, elbows out to the sides, and a dumbbell in each hand, held level with your chest, inhale, and then exhale as you press the dumbbells toward the ceiling. Hold at the top, and then return to the start position. Do not relax arms on the stability ball; keep elbows extended out to your sides. (See photos 25a and 25b above.)

Intermediate: Chest Press over Stability Ball, Alternating Arms

Same position as the Basic, except you will perform the exercise by alternating arms through the movement.

Advanced: One-Arm Chest Press over Stability Ball with Rotation

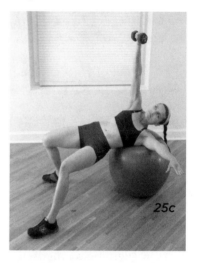

Same as the Basic, except you will use only one arm with a dumbbell, and press the dumbbell toward the ceiling as you roll onto your opposite shoulder. Hold and repeat for the desired number of repetitions. Then, with dumbbell in the opposite hand, perform the movement with that arm. Rotate torso while you perform this movement and keep other arm straight out to the side. (See photo 25c, right.)

25c

Sets/Reps: Off-Season—three sets of 8 to 12 reps

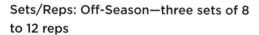

3. Jump Squats onto Step or Box

Purpose: To strengthen glutes, hamstrings, quads, ankles, abs, core, and balance.

Basic: Jump Squats onto Step or Box

Start in a standing position with your feet about shoulder-width apart in front of a step or box. With your arms at your sides, inhale and perform a deep squat. From the deep squat position, exhale and jump onto the step

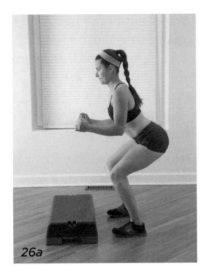
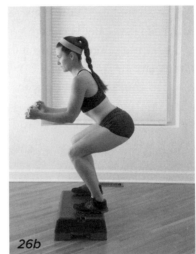

26a
26b

or box with both feet and land in a squat position. Step off step or box and repeat the squat and jump. (See photos 26a and 26b above.)

Intermediate: Jump Squats onto BOSU

Same as the Basic, except you will start by standing in front of a BOSU, jumping onto it, and landing in a squat position. Step off the BOSU and perform the squat and jump again.

Advanced: Jump Squats on the BOSU

Start by standing on the BOSU. Perform a deep squat and jump by extending your legs, hips, and glutes straight up, then landing in a deep squat position back on the BOSU. Repeat the jump and squat.

Sets/Reps: Off-Season—three sets of 8 to 12 reps

4. Side Lunge with Front Raise

Purpose: To strengthen glutes, hamstrings, quads, ab/adductors, shoulders, and core.

Basic: Side Lunge with Front Raise

Start in a standing position with a dumbbell in each hand at your sides. Perform a side lunge, keeping your hips back and lunging leg bent while your other leg stays straight. From that position raise your arms with dumbbells out straight to shoulder height, hold, and then simultaneously bring your arms back to your sides while extending your hips, glutes, and quads back to the start position. Perform half of the repetitions on one leg and then switch and perform half of the repetitions on the other leg. (See page 35.)

Intermediate: Side Lunge onto Step with Front Raise

Same as the Basic, except side-lunge onto a step.

Advanced: Side Lunge onto BOSU with One-Arm Front Raise

Same as the Intermediate, except side-lunge onto a BOSU so your foot strikes the center of it, and raise the same side arm. Then, repeat with other leg and arm.

Sets/Reps: Off-Season—three sets of 8 to 12 reps / Advanced—three sets of 8 to 12 reps each side

5. Obliques over BOSU

Purpose: To strengthen obliques.

Basic: Obliques over BOSU

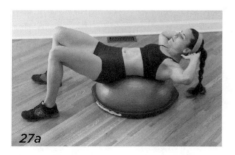
27a
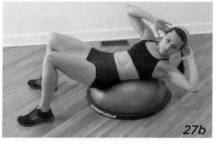
27b

Start by lying on the BOSU with the small of your back centered on top, both arms behind your head, and your feet on the floor. Slightly raise your torso off the BOSU while pointing one elbow toward the opposite knee. Hold and return to the start position and then repeat with the opposite elbow toward the other knee. Repeat by alternating sides. (See photos 27a and 27b above.)

Intermediate: Obliques over BOSU with One Leg Raised

Same as the Basic, except with both hands behind your head, slightly raise your torso while raising the left leg and pointing the right elbow toward the left knee. Outstretched leg should remain off the floor. Repeat on that side and then switch legs and repeat on the other side. (See photo 27c above.)

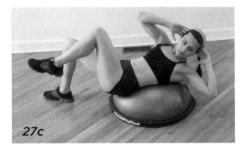
27c

Advanced: Bicycles over BOSU with Legs Raised

Same as the Intermediate, except with both hands behind your head, raise your torso and legs off the floor so you are balanced on the BOSU. Extend one leg straight and keep the other leg bent. Start the movement by bringing the knee of the extended leg to the opposite elbow so they make con-

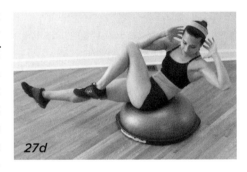
27d

tact. Repeat this movement with the opposite arm and leg, alternating the movement from one side to the other while maintaining balance on the BOSU. (See photo 27d above.)

Sets/Reps: Off-Season—three sets of 8 to 12 reps

Second Phase: Preseason of Short-Course Triathlete Program (reps increase to 10–12 range)

Once we are about eight to twelve weeks away from our first major race of the year, we will transition into the Preseason Phase of the Short-Course Triathlete Program. This phase starts with the Fink Five and then goes right into the following three exercises, which most practiced athletes can complete in about 7.5 minutes. If an athlete starts with the Easy Eight warm-up routine (5 minutes), then completes the Fink Five (12 minutes), and then finishes up with the following three Preseason Exercises (7.5 minutes), he or she can complete the entire Preseason Program in less than 25 minutes.

1. Lateral Lunge/Squat across BOSU

Purpose: To strengthen glutes, hamstrings, quads, ankles, core, and balance, and to develop power.

Basic: Lateral Lunge/Squat across BOSU

Start by standing on the BOSU. Then, take one leg and lunge to the side into a deep squat, keeping your other foot on the BOSU. Then, quickly jump your off foot onto the BOSU and lunge with the other leg to the opposite side. Repeat side to side quickly while maintaining good form. (See page 39.)

Intermediate: Lateral Lunge/Squat across BOSU with Medicine Ball Reach

Start by standing on the BOSU with a medicine ball at chest height, with bent arms. Take one leg and lunge to the side into a deep squat, keeping your other foot on the BOSU, and simultaneously extend the medicine ball straight out in front. Bring the medicine ball back to your chest, and then quickly jump your off foot onto the BOSU and lunge with the other leg to the opposite side while reaching out front again with the medicine ball. Repeat side to side quickly while maintaining good form.

Advanced: Lateral Lunge/Squat across BOSU with 180° Turn

Start by standing on the BOSU. Take one leg and lunge to the side into a deep squat, keeping the other foot on the BOSU. Then, quickly jump straight up with both legs and simultaneously make a 180° turn so you face the opposite direction, landing with the opposite foot on the BOSU and the other foot on the ground. Jump across the BOSU and repeat 180° turn on that side. Repeat side to side quickly with the 180° turn while maintaining good form. (See page 40.)

Sets/Reps: Preseason—three sets of 10 to 12 reps

2. One-Leg Press to Hop (with or without dumbbells)

Purpose: To strengthen glutes, hamstrings, quads, ankles, core, and balance, and to develop power.

Basic: One-Leg Press with Foot on Step (with or without dumbbells)

Start by standing in a lunge position with one foot on the step and the other foot behind, with knee bent almost to the floor. Perform a one-leg press with the leg on the step and rise to a standing position while bringing the opposite leg up with raised knee. Return to the start position and repeat on that leg and then switch to the other leg. (See page 40.)

Intermediate: One-Leg Press to Hop with Foot on Step (with or without dumbbells)

Same as the Basic, except after you complete the press, hop on the same leg while keeping the opposite leg raised in a chair pose. Return to the start position and repeat on the same leg before switching to the opposite leg for the remaining repetitions. (See page 41.)

Advanced: One-Leg Press to Hop with Foot on BOSU (with or without dumbbells)

Same as the Intermediate, except start with one foot on the BOSU. Then, after you complete the press, hop on that same leg while raising the opposite knee in a chair pose. Repeat on the same leg before switching to the opposite leg.

Sets/Reps: Preseason—three sets of 10 to 12 reps, each leg

3. Get-ups off BOSU with Arms at Your Sides

Purpose: To strengthen core and abdominals, glutes, quads, and hamstrings.

Basic: Get-ups off the BOSU with Arms at Your Sides

Start by sitting on the BOSU with arms at your sides and bent knees. Extend your torso back so you are completely parallel to the floor and legs are raised off the floor. Then, raise torso and simultaneously put your feet on the floor and stand straight up. Then, return to the start position and repeat. (See page 41.)

Intermediate: Get-ups off BOSU with Arms Raised

Same as the Basic, except with both arms extended over your head for the entire exercise. Raise your torso and simultaneously bring your feet to the floor and stand up, keeping arms extended over your head.

Advanced: Get-ups off the Floor with Medicine Ball Overhead

Same as the Intermediate, except start by lying on the floor instead of the BOSU, with knees bent and holding a medicine ball over your head. As you begin to "get up," bring the ball down from over your head to in front of your chest.

Sets/Reps: Preseason—three sets of 10 to 12 reps

Third Phase: Competitive Season of Short-Course Triathlete Program (reps increase to 15–20 range)

Once we have completed our first major race of the year, we will transition into the Competitive-Season Phase of the Short-Course Triathlete Program. This phase starts with the Fink Five and then goes right into the following three exercises, which most practiced athletes can complete in about 5 minutes. If an athlete starts with the Easy Eight warm-up routine (5 minutes), then completes the Fink Five (12 minutes), and then finishes up with the following three Competitive-Season Exercises (7.5 minutes), he or she can complete the entire Competitive-Season Program in less than 25 minutes. Additional Note: As part of a proper pre-race taper, it is our general suggestion not to perform strength training during the week immediately preceding a major race.

1. Rear Deltoid Flys in Stork Position

Purpose: To strengthen deltoids, rhomboids, hamstrings, quads, core, and balance.

Basic: Rear Deltoid Flys in Stork Position

Start in a standing position with a dumbbell in each hand. Raise one leg straight behind you and balance on the other leg in a stork position, letting your arms hang straight down. Depress your shoulder blades toward your spine and raise the dumbbells with slightly bent arms out to the sides, but not higher than shoulder height. Hold for a 2-second count and then return arms back to the start position and repeat. Keep hands soft as you squeeze your shoulder blades together to elevate the weights. Perform half the repetitions on one leg and then switch and perform half the repetitions on the other leg. (See page 36.)

Intermediate: Rear Deltoid Flys in Stork Position, Alternating Arms

Same as the Basic, except perform this exercise by raising one arm at a time and alternating arms. Perform half of the repetitions on one leg and then switch and perform half of the repetitions on the other leg.

Advanced: Rear Deltoid Flys with One-Leg Squat in Stork Position

Same as the Basic, except start this exercise from the stork position and begin with a one-leg squat; then, as you extend from the squat, simultaneously raise the weights as you return to the start position. Perform half of the repetitions on one leg and then switch and perform half of the repetitions on the other leg.

Sets/Reps: Competitive Season—three sets of 12 to 15 reps

2. Superman on BOSU

Purpose: To strengthen back, shoulders, glutes, hamstrings, abdominals, and core.

Basic: Superman on BOSU

Start by lying facedown with your hips centered on the BOSU, your legs straight and hip-width apart, and your palms facing up. Extend your shoulder blades back and down toward your spine. Inhale to prepare for the movement and then exhale as you extend your lower back, squeezing your glutes as you extend your torso up while rotating your thumbs toward the ceiling. Hold for one second in that position before returning to the start position. (See page 44.)

Intermediate: Superman on BOSU with Arms Overhead

Same as the Basic, except raise your arms over your head and perform the movement without rotating your thumbs toward the ceiling. (See page 44.)

Advanced: Swimming on BOSU

Start by lying facedown, balanced on your midsection over the BOSU, with legs extended and arms overhead. Raise your arms and legs off the floor, find your balance, and then perform a swimming-type movement (no need to do the crawl stroke, exactly) by fluttering your arms and legs for about 30 to 60 seconds. (See page 44.)

Sets/Reps: Competitive Season—three sets of 12 to 15 reps
Advanced: Sets/Reps: Competitive Season—three sets of 30 to 60 seconds

3. Overhead Raises with Stretch Cords or Bands

Purpose: To strengthen shoulders, back, lats, abdominals, and core.

Basic: Overhead Raises with Stretch Cords or Bands

Start by holding one end of a stretch cord in both hands and place your foot on the other end of the stretch cord on the floor to hold it in place. Give yourself enough slack so you can extend the stretch cord directly over your head, keeping your arms straight. While keeping your arms straight, raise the stretch cord directly above your shoulders and head; then, lower to start position and repeat.

Intermediate: Overhead Raises with Stretch Cords or Bands in Lunge Position

Same as the Basic, except stagger your feet in a lunge position while raising the stretch cord directly over your head. Split the repetitions between each leg. (See page 45.)

Advanced: Squat with Overhead Raises Using Kettle Bell

Start by standing with feet shoulder-width apart, holding one kettle bell with both hands. Begin by squatting back and bringing the kettle bell through your legs. Then, while extending out of the squat and returning to a standing position, simultaneously swing the kettle bell straight out in front and above your head while keeping your arms straight. Then, slowly lower the kettle bell and return to the start position. (See page 46.)

Sets/Reps: Competitive Season—three sets of 12 to 15 reps

Runners—Road Racer Program

(5K Road Races to Full Marathon)

This program includes the following exercises:

Off-Season	Preseason	Competitive Season
Fink Five	Fink Five	Fink Five
1. Dumbbell Arm Swings	1. Lateral Lunge	1. Get-ups off BOSU
2. Squat with Ax Chop	2. One-Leg Press/	2. Overhead Raises
3. Jump Squats	Hop	3. Superman on BOSU
4. Dead Lifts with	3. Obliques over	
Dumbbells	BOSU	
5. Ab Triangles		

First Phase: Off-Season of Runners—Road Racer Program

In the Off-Season, the Runners—Road Racer Program starts with the Fink Five and then goes right into the following five exercises, which most practiced athletes can complete in 12 minutes. If an athlete starts with the Easy Eight warm-up routine (5 minutes), then completes the Fink Five (12 minutes), and then finishes up with the following five exercises (12 minutes), he or she can complete the entire Off-Season Program in less than 30 minutes.

1. Dumbbell Arm Swings

Purpose: To strengthen pectorals, shoulders, glutes, arms, abdominals, and core.

Basic: Dumbbell Arm Swings

Start by standing in a staggered-step position with feet about 12 inches apart, holding a dumbbell in each hand. With good posture, chest out and belly in, raise weights by bending at your elbows and keeping forearms mostly parallel to the ground, as shown in photo 28a. Simultaneously, pull one elbow straight back so your hand is underneath your armpit and other arm/elbow

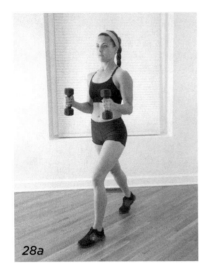
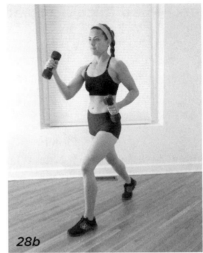

28a

28b

is forward, as in a running motion. Swing shoulders back and forth, maintaining good upright posture and pulling shoulders back. Reverse foot position halfway through the repetitions. (See photos 28a and 28b above.)

Intermediate: Arm Swings with Stretch Cord

Same position as the Basic, except you will hold the ends of the stretch cord in each hand. Secure the stretch cord in a doorjamb so that you have two equidistant ends to the cord. Maintain a staggered position for half the number of repetitions, then switch staggered position with opposite leg and perform the remaining number of repetitions.

Advanced: Arm Swings with Stretch Cord Standing with Leg Raised

Same as the Intermediate, except you will stand on one leg with the other knee raised in front. Perform half the number of repetitions on one leg and then repeat the remaining number of repetitions on the opposite leg.

Sets/Reps: Off-Season—three sets of 8 to 12 reps

2. Squat with Ax Chop on BOSU

Purpose: To strengthen hamstrings, quads, glutes, abdominals, arms, shoulders, core, and back.

Basic: Squat with Ax Chop on BOSU Using Medicine Ball

Start by standing on top of the BOSU, holding a medicine ball at shoulder height to one side, with arms bent. As you are performing a squat, and at the same pace as the squat, lower the medicine ball to the opposite side across your body in a chopping motion until you complete the squat. Return to the start position, extending the legs while reversing the chopping motion, and then repeat on the same side before switching to the other side. (See page 33.)

Intermediate: Squat with Ax Chop on BOSU Using Kettle Bell

Same as the Basic, except use a kettle bell to perform the exercise.

Advanced: Side Lunge with Ax Chop on BOSU Using Kettle Bell

Start by standing on top of the BOSU, holding a kettle bell at shoulder height to one side, with arms bent. As you are performing a side lunge, swing the kettle bell to the opposite side across your body in a chopping motion to the outside of your lunging leg until you complete the lunge. Return to the start position and bring the kettle bell back to the opposite shoulder by reversing the chopping motion. Repeat on the opposite side.

Sets/Reps: Off-Season—three sets of 8 to 12 reps, each side

3. Jump Squats onto Step or Box

Purpose: To strengthen glutes, hamstrings, quads, ankles, abs, core, and balance.

Basic: Jump Squats onto Step or Box

Start in a standing position with your feet about shoulder-width apart in front of a step or box. With your arms at your sides, inhale and perform a deep squat. From the deep squat position, exhale and jump onto the step or box with both feet, landing in a squat position. Step off step or box and repeat the squat and jump. (See page 50.)

Intermediate: Jump Squats onto BOSU

Same as the Basic, except you will start by standing in front of a BOSU, jumping onto it and landing in a squat position. Step off the BOSU and perform the squat and jump again.

Advanced: Jump Squats on the BOSU

Start by standing on the BOSU. Perform a deep squat and jump by extending your legs, hips, and glutes straight up and then landing in a deep squat position back on the BOSU. Repeat the jump and squat.

Sets/Reps: Off-Season—three sets of 8 to 12 reps

4. Dead Lifts with Dumbbells

Purpose: To strengthen glutes, hamstrings, quads, ab/adductors, calves, and core.

Basic: Dead Lifts with Dumbbells

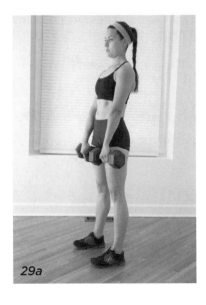
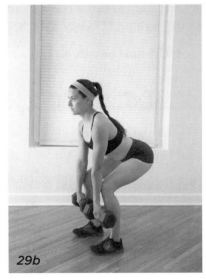

29a   29b

Start in a standing position with feet about shoulder-width apart and a dumbbell in each hand. Keep belly drawn in and shoulder blades back and down. Keeping arms straight down the entire time, lower the dumbbells toward the floor, with knees slightly bent and a straight back. Then return to a standing position by pushing through your glutes and hamstrings as you return to the start position. (See photos 29a and 29b above.)

Intermediate: Dead Lifts with Dumbbells to Calf Raise

Same as the Basic, except as you return to start position from dead lift, go immediately onto your toes and perform a calf raise. Be sure to maintain good posture, back flat and lifting through your glutes and hamstrings. (See photo 29c, right.)

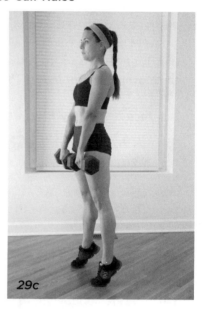

29c

Advanced: Dead Lifts with Dumbbells to Calf Raise on One Leg

Same as the Intermediate, except you will perform the dead lift to calf raise while standing on one leg only. Be sure to maintain good posture, drawing your belly in and keeping your shoulders back and down. You can keep your off leg straight or slightly bent.

Sets/Reps: Off-Season—three sets of 8 to 12 reps

5. Abs—Open-and-Close Triangles

Purpose: To strengthen overall core and abdominals.

Basic: Abs—Open-and-Close Triangles

Start by lying on the floor on your back with legs extended straight so they are perpendicular to the floor and your arms extended toward your knees. Your legs, torso, and arms should almost form a right triangle. Simultaneously, lower your legs together toward the floor and your arms straight over your head from your shoulders. Hold your position when you are straight but not quite touching the ground, and then return to the start position and repeat. (See page 37.)

Intermediate: Abs—Stability Ball Pass from Hands to Feet

Same as the Basic, except you start with a stability ball in your hands as you lower your arms overhead and your legs toward the floor. Then, simultaneously, raise your arms and legs together and pass the stability ball from your hands to between your feet and repeat the movement. Continue passing the ball from your hands to your feet at each return to starting point and make the movement continuous. (See page 38.)

Advanced: Stability Ball Pass from Hands to Feet with Raised Torso

Same as the Intermediate, except raise your torso off the floor every time you raise your arms back to the straight position, with or without the stability ball.

Sets/Reps: Off-Season—three sets of 8 to 12 reps

Second Phase: Preseason of Runners—Road Racer Program (reps increase to 10–12 range)

Once we are about eight to twelve weeks away from our first major race of the year, we will transition into the Preseason Phase of the Runners–Road Racer Program. This phase starts with the Fink Five and then goes right into the following three exercises, which most practiced athletes can complete in about 7.5 minutes. If an athlete starts with the Easy Eight warm-up routine (5 minutes), then completes the Fink Five (12 minutes), and then finishes up with the following three Preseason Exercises (7.5 minutes), he or she can complete the entire Preseason Program in less than 25 minutes.

1. Lateral Lunge/Squat across BOSU

Purpose: To strengthen glutes, hamstrings, quads, ankles, core, and balance, and to develop power.

Basic: Lateral Lunge/Squat across BOSU

Start by standing on the BOSU. Then, take one leg and lunge to the side into a deep squat, keeping your other foot on the BOSU. Then quickly jump your off foot onto the BOSU and lunge with the other leg to the opposite side. Repeat side to side quickly while maintaining good form. (See page 39.)

Intermediate: Lateral Lunge/Squat across BOSU with Medicine Ball Reach

Start by standing on the BOSU with a medicine ball at chest height, with bent arms. Take one leg and lunge to the side into a deep squat, keeping your other foot on the BOSU, and simultaneously extend the medicine ball straight out in front. Bring the medicine ball back to your chest, and then quickly jump your off foot onto the BOSU and lunge with the other leg to the opposite side while reaching out front again with the medicine ball. Repeat side to side quickly while maintaining good form.

Advanced: Lateral Lunge/Squat across BOSU with 180° Turn

Start by standing on the BOSU. Take one leg and lunge to the side into a deep squat, keeping the other foot on the BOSU. Then quickly jump straight up with both legs and simultaneously make a 180° turn so you face the opposite direction, landing with the opposite foot on the BOSU and the other foot on the ground. Jump across the BOSU and repeat 180° turn on that side. Repeat side to side quickly with the 180° turn while maintaining good form. (See page 40.)

Sets/Reps: Preseason—three sets of 10 to 12 reps

2. One-Leg Press to Hop (with or without dumbbells)

Purpose: To strengthen glutes, hamstrings, quads, ankles, core, and balance, and to develop power.

Basic: One-Leg Press with Foot on Step (with or without dumbbells)

Start by standing in a lunge position with one foot on the step and the other foot behind, with knee bent almost to the floor. Perform a one-leg press with the leg on the step and rise to a standing position while bringing the opposite leg up with raised knee. Return to the start position and repeat on that leg and then switch to the other leg. (See page 40.)

Intermediate: One-Leg Press to Hop with Foot on Step (with or without dumbbells)

Same as the Basic, except after you complete the press, hop on the same leg while keeping the opposite leg raised in a chair pose. Return to the start position and repeat on the same leg before switching to the opposite leg for the remaining repetitions. (See page 41.)

Advanced: One-Leg Press to Hop with Foot on BOSU (with or without dumbbells)

Same as the Intermediate, except start with one foot on the BOSU. Then, after you complete the press, hop on that same leg while raising the opposite knee in a chair pose. Repeat on the same leg before switching to the opposite leg.

Sets/Reps: Preseason—three sets of 10 to 12 reps, each leg

3. Obliques over BOSU

Purpose: To strengthen obliques.

Basic: Obliques over BOSU

Start by lying on the BOSU with the small of your back centered on top, both arms behind your head, and your feet on the floor. Slightly raise your torso off the BOSU while pointing one elbow toward the opposite knee. Hold and return to the start position and then repeat with the opposite elbow toward the other knee. Repeat by alternating sides. (See page 51.)

Intermediate: Obliques over BOSU with One Leg Raised

Same as the Basic, except with both hands behind your head, slightly raise your torso while raising the left leg and pointing the right elbow toward the left knee. Outstretched leg should remain off the floor. Repeat on that side and then switch legs and repeat on the other side. (See page 52).

Advanced: Bicycles over BOSU with Legs Raised

Same as the Intermediate, except with both hands behind your head, raise your torso and legs off the floor so you are balanced on the BOSU. Extend one leg straight and keep the other leg bent. Start the movement by bringing the knee of the extended leg to the opposite elbow so they make contact. Repeat this movement with the opposite arm and leg alternating the movement from one side to the other while maintaining balance on the BOSU. (See page 52.)

Sets/Reps: Preseason—three sets of 10 to 12 reps

Third Phase: Competitive Season of Runners—Road Racer Program (reps increase to 12–15 range)

Once we have completed our first major race of the year, we will transition into the Competitive-Season Phase of the Runners—Road Racer Program. This phase starts with the Fink Five and then goes right into the following three exercises, which most practiced athletes can complete in about 7.5 minutes. If an athlete starts with the Easy Eight warm-up routine (5 minutes), then completes the Fink Five (12 minutes), and then finishes up with the following three Competitive-Season Exercises (7.5 minutes), he or she can complete the entire Competitive-Season Program in less than 25 minutes. Additional Note: As part of a proper pre-race taper, it is our general suggestion not to perform strength training during the week immediately preceding a major race.

1. Get-ups off BOSU with Arms at Your Sides

Purpose: To strengthen core and abdominals, glutes, quads, and hamstrings.

Basic: Get-ups off the BOSU with Arms at Your Sides

Start by sitting on the BOSU with arms at your sides and bent knees. Extend your torso back so you are completely parallel to the floor and legs are raised off the floor. Then, raise torso and simultaneously put your feet on the floor and stand straight up. Then, return to the start position and repeat. (See page 41.)

Intermediate: Get-ups off BOSU with Arms Raised

Same as the Basic, except with both arms extended over your head for the entire exercise. Raise your torso and simultaneously bring your feet to the floor and stand up, keeping arms extended over your head.

Advanced: Get-ups off Floor with Medicine Ball Overhead

Same as the Intermediate, except start by lying on the floor instead of the BOSU, with knees bent and holding a medicine ball over your head. As you begin to "get up," bring the ball down from over your head to in front of your chest.

Sets/Reps: Competitive Season—three sets of 12 to 15 reps

2. Overhead Raises with Stretch Cords or Bands

Purpose: To strengthen shoulders, back, lats, abdominals, and core.

Basic: Overhead Raises with Stretch Cords or Bands

Start by holding one end of a stretch cord in both hands, placing your foot on the other end of the stretch cord on the floor to hold it in place. Give yourself enough slack so you can extend the stretch cord directly over your head, keeping your arms straight. While keeping your arms straight, raise the stretch cord directly above your shoulders and head; then, lower to start position and repeat. (See page 45.)

Intermediate: Overhead Raises with Stretch Cords or Bands in Lunge Position

Same as the Basic, except stagger your feet in a lunge position while raising the stretch cord directly over your head. Split the repetitions between each leg.

Advanced: Squat with Overhead Raises Using Kettle Bell

Start by standing with feet shoulder-width apart, holding one kettle bell with both hands. Begin by squatting back and bringing the kettle bell through

your legs. Then, while extending out of the squat and returning to a standing position, simultaneously swing the kettle bell straight out in front and above your head while keeping your arms straight. Then, slowly lower the kettle bell and return to the start position. (See page 46.)

Sets/Reps: Competitive Season—three sets of 12 to 15 reps

3. Superman on BOSU

Purpose: To strengthen back, shoulders, glutes, hamstrings, abdominals, and core.

Basic: Superman on BOSU

Start by lying facedown with your hips centered on the BOSU, your legs straight and hip-width apart, and your palms facing up. Extend your shoulder blades back and down toward your spine. Inhale to prepare for the movement and then exhale as you extend your lower back, squeezing your glutes as you extend your torso up while rotating your thumbs toward the ceiling. Hold for 1 second in that position before returning to the start position. (See page 44.)

Intermediate: Superman on BOSU with Arms Overhead

Same as the Basic, except raise your arms over your head and perform the movement without rotating your thumbs toward the ceiling. (See page 44.)

Advanced: Swimming on BOSU

Start by lying facedown, balanced on your midsection over the BOSU, with legs extended and arms overhead. Raise your arms and legs off the floor, find your balance, and then perform a swimming-type movement (no need to do the crawl stroke, exactly) by fluttering your arms and legs for about 30 to 60 seconds. (See page 44.)

Sets/Reps: Competitive Season—three sets of 12 to 15 reps
Advanced: Sets/Reps: Competitive Season—three sets of 30 to 60 seconds

Runners—Ultra Distance Program

(50K to 100-Mile Ultras)

This program includes the following exercises:

Off-Season	Preseason	Competitive Season
Fink Five	Fink Five	Fink Five
1. Ax Chop on BOSU	1. Squat, Curl, and Press	1. Get-ups off BOSU
2. Dumbbell Arm Swings	2. One-Leg Press/Hop	2. Overhead Raises
3. Dead Lifts with Dumbbells	3. Side Planks	3. Superman on BOSU
4. Side Lunge with Front Raise		
5. Ab Triangles		

First Phase: Off-Season of Runners—Ultra Distance Program

In the Off-Season, the Runners—Ultra Distance Program starts with the Fink Five and then goes right into the following five exercises, which most practiced athletes can complete in 12 minutes. If an athlete starts with the Easy Eight warm-up routine (5 minutes), then completes the Fink Five (12 minutes), and then finishes up with the following five exercises (12 minutes), he or she can complete the program in less than 30 minutes.

1. Squat with Ax Chop on BOSU

Purpose: To strengthen hamstrings, quads, glutes, abdominals, arms, shoulders, and back.

Basic: Squat with Ax Chop on BOSU Using Medicine Ball

Start by standing on top of the BOSU and holding a medicine ball at shoulder height to one side, with arms bent. As you are performing a squat, and at the same pace as the squat, lower the medicine ball to the opposite side across your body in a chopping motion until you complete the squat. Return to the start position, extending the legs while reversing the chopping motion, and then repeat on the same side before switching to the other side. (See page 33.)

Intermediate: Squat with Ax Chop on BOSU Using Kettle Bell

Same as the Basic, except use a kettle bell to perform the exercise.

Advanced: Side Lunge with Ax Chop on BOSU Using Kettle Bell

Start by standing on top of the BOSU and holding a kettle bell at shoulder height to one side, with arms bent. As you are performing a side lunge, swing the kettle bell to the opposite side across your body in a chopping motion to the outside of your lunging leg until you complete the lunge. Return to the start position and bring the kettle bell back to the opposite shoulder by reversing the chopping motion. Repeat on the opposite side.

Sets/Reps: Off-Season—three sets of 8 to 12 reps, each side

2. Dumbbell Arm Swings

Purpose: To strengthen pectorals, shoulders, glutes, arms, abdominals, and core.

Basic: Dumbbell Arm Swings

Start by standing in a staggered-step position with feet about 12 inches apart, holding a dumbbell in each hand. With good posture, chest out and belly in, raise weights by bending at your elbows and keeping forearms mostly parallel to the ground, as shown in photo 28a. Simultaneously, pull one elbow straight back so your hand is underneath your armpit and other arm/elbow is forward, as in a running motion. Swing shoulders back and forth, maintaining good upright posture and pulling shoulders back. Reverse foot position halfway through the repetitions. (See page 60.)

Intermediate: Arm Swings with Stretch Cord

Same position as the Basic, except you will hold the ends of the stretch cord in each hand. Secure the stretch cord in a doorjamb so that you have two equidistant ends to the cord. Maintain a staggered position for half the number of repetitions, then switch staggered position with opposite leg and perform the remaining number of repetitions.

Advanced: Arm Swings with Stretch Cord Standing with Leg Raised

Same as the Intermediate, except you will stand on one leg with the other knee raised in front. Perform half the number of repetitions on one leg and then repeat the remaining number of repetitions on the opposite leg.

Sets/Reps: Off-Season—three sets of 8 to 12 reps

3. Dead Lifts with Dumbbells

Purpose: To strengthen glutes, hamstrings, quads, ab/adductors, calves, and core.

Basic: Dead Lifts with Dumbbells

Start in a standing position with feet about shoulder-width apart and a dumbbell in each hand. Keep belly drawn in and shoulder blades back and down. Keeping arms straight down the entire time, lower the dumbbells toward the floor with knees slightly bent and a straight back. Then return to a standing position by pushing through your glutes and hamstrings as you return to the start position. (See page 62.)

Intermediate: Dead Lifts with Dumbbells to Calf Raise

Same as the Basic, except as you return to start position from dead lift, go immediately onto your toes and perform a calf raise. Be sure to maintain good posture, back flat and lifting through your glutes and hamstrings. (See page 63.)

Advanced: Dead Lifts with Dumbbells to Calf Raise on One Leg

Same as the Intermediate, except you will perform the dead lift to calf raise while standing on one leg only. Be sure to maintain good posture, drawing your belly in and keeping your shoulders back and down. You can keep your off leg straight or slightly bent.

Sets/Reps: Off-Season—three sets of 8 to 12 reps

4. Side Lunge with Front Raise

Purpose: To strengthen glutes, hamstrings, quads, ab/adductors, shoulders, and core.

Basic: Side Lunge with Front Raise

Start in a standing position with a dumbbell in each hand at your sides. Perform a side lunge, keeping your hips back and lunging leg bent while your other leg stays straight. From that position raise your arms with dumbbells out straight to shoulder height, hold, and then simultaneously bring your arms back to your sides while extending your hips, glutes, and quads back to the start position. Perform half of the repetitions on one leg and then switch and perform half of the repetitions on the other leg. (See page 35.)

Intermediate: Side Lunge onto Step with Front Raise

Same as the Basic, except side-lunge onto a step.

Advanced: Side Lunge onto BOSU with One-Arm Front Raise

Same as the Intermediate, except side-lunge onto a BOSU so your foot strikes the center of it, and raise the same side arm. Then, repeat with other leg and arm.

Sets/Reps: Off-Season—three sets of 8 to 12 reps / Advanced—three sets of 8 to 12 reps, each side

5. Abs—Open-and-Close Triangles

Purpose: To strengthen overall core and abdominals.

Basic: Abs—Open-and-Close Triangles

Start by lying on the floor on your back with legs extended straight so they are perpendicular to the floor and your arms extended toward your knees. Your legs, torso, and arms should almost form a right triangle. Simultaneously, lower your legs together toward the floor and your arms straight over your head from your shoulders. Hold your position when you are straight but not quite touching the ground, and then return to the start position and repeat. (See page 37.)

Intermediate: Abs—Stability Ball Pass from Hands to Feet

Same as the Basic, except you start with a stability ball in your hands as you lower your arms overhead and your legs toward the floor. Then, simultaneously, raise your arms and legs together and pass the stability ball from your hands to between your feet and repeat the movement. Continue passing the ball from your hands to your feet at each return to starting point and make the movement continuous. (See page 38.)

Advanced: Stability Ball Pass from Hands to Feet with Raised Torso

Same as the Intermediate, except raise your torso off the floor every time you raise your arms back to the straight position, with or without the stability ball.

Sets/Reps: Off-Season—three sets of 8 to 12 reps

Second Phase: Preseason of Runners—Ultra Distance Program (reps increase to 10–15 range)

Once we are about eight to twelve weeks away from our first major race of the year, we will transition into the Preseason Phase of the Runners—Ultra Distance Program. This phase starts with the Fink Five and then goes right into the following three exercises, which most practiced athletes can complete in about 7.5 minutes. If an athlete starts with the Easy Eight warm-up routine (5 minutes), then completes the Fink Five (12 minutes), and then finishes up with the following three Preseason Exercises (7.5 minutes), he or she can complete the entire Preseason Program in less than 25 minutes.

1. Squat to Curl and Press

Purpose: To strengthen glutes, hamstrings, biceps, shoulders, and core.

Basic: Squat to Curl and Press

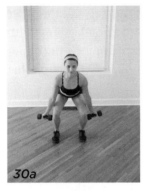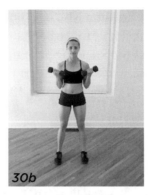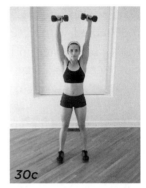

Start in a standing position with a dumbbell in each hand. Begin by inhaling, and then perform a freestanding squat. As you return from the squat position, begin to curl the dumbbells as you get to the start position and then press the dumbbells over your head. Return the dumbbells to your sides and repeat. (See photos 30a, 30b, and 30c above.)

Intermediate: Squat on BOSU, Curl and Press

Same as the Basic, except start by standing on the BOSU.

Advanced: Squat on One Leg, Curl and Press

Same as the Basic, except start by raising one leg straight up, with knee bent and parallel to the ground. Swing leg back, perform squat with other leg, then curl and press the weights over your head, and then return the weights to your sides. Repeat with same leg through a complete set of repetitions before switching to the other leg.

Sets/Reps: Preseason—three sets of 10 to 12 reps

2. One-Leg Press to Hop (with or without dumbbells)

Purpose: To strengthen glutes, hamstrings, quads, ankles, core, and balance, and to develop power.

Basic: One-Leg Press with Foot on Step (with or without dumbbells)

Start by standing in a lunge position with one foot on the step and the other foot behind, with knee bent almost to the floor. Perform a one-leg press with the leg on the step and raise to a standing position while bringing the opposite leg up with raised knee. Return to the start position and repeat on that leg and then switch to the other leg. (See page 40.)

Intermediate: One-Leg Press to Hop with Foot on Step (with or without dumbbells)

Same as the Basic, except after you complete the press, hop on the same leg while keeping the opposite leg raised in a chair pose. Return to the start position and repeat on the same leg before switching to the opposite leg for the remaining repetitions. (See photo 20c on page 41.)

Advanced: One-Leg Press to Hop with Foot on BOSU (with or without dumbbells)

Same as the Intermediate, except start with one foot on the BOSU. Then, after you complete the press, hop on that same leg while raising the opposite knee in a chair pose. Repeat on the same leg before switching to the opposite leg.

Sets/Reps: Preseason—three sets of 10 to 12 reps

3. Side Planks

Purpose: To strengthen obliques, abdominals, core, and shoulders.

Basic: Side Plank on Floor

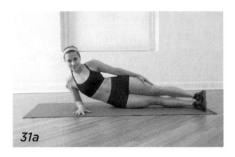
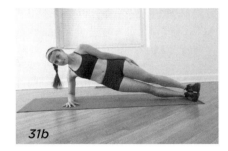

31a   31b

Start by lying on your side on the floor, with your upper body resting on your bent elbow under your shoulder and your other arm at your side. Draw in your belly and hold while raising your hip and torso off the floor, with weight on your forearm, until there is a straight line from your ankles to your head. Hold for a 5- to 10-second count and maintain drawn-in belly as you lower hips to the floor. Repeat on your other side. (See photos 31a and 31b above.)

Intermediate: Side Plank on Floor with Arm Raise

Same as the Basic, except raise and lower your top arm repeatedly, with palm facing up while holding the position for a 15- to 30-second count, and then repeat on your other side.

Advanced: Side Plank on Floor with Ab Crunch

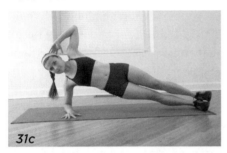 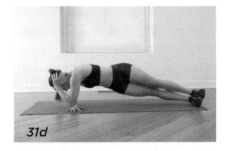

Same as the Basic, except place the hand of your top arm behind your head with bent elbow. While holding plank position, rotate your elbow toward the floor and repeat for the desired number of repetitions, and then repeat on your other side. (See photos 31c and 31d above.)

Sets/Reps: Preseason—three sets of 10 to 12 reps, each side

Third Phase: Competitive Season of Runners—Ultra Distance Program (reps increase to 12–15 range)

Once we have completed our first major race of the year, we will transition into the Competitive-Season Phase of the Runners—Ultra Distance Program. This phase starts with the Fink Five and then goes right into the following three exercises, which most practiced athletes can complete in about 7.5 minutes. If an athlete starts with the Easy Eight warm-up routine (5 minutes), then completes the Fink Five (12 minutes), and then finishes up with the following three Competitive-Season Exercises (7.5 minutes), he or she can complete the entire Competitive-Season Program in less than 25 minutes. Additional Note: As part of a proper pre-race taper, it is our general suggestion not to perform strength training during the week immediately preceding a major race.

1. Get-ups off BOSU with Arms at Your Sides

Purpose: To strengthen core and abdominals, glutes, quads, and hamstrings.

Basic: Get-ups off the BOSU with Arms at Your Sides

Start by sitting on the BOSU with arms at your sides and bent knees. Extend your torso back so you are completely parallel to the floor and legs are raised off the floor. Then, raise torso and simultaneously put your feet on the floor and stand straight up. Then, return to the start position and repeat. (See photos 21a, 21b, and 21c on page 41.)

Intermediate: Get-ups off BOSU with Arms Raised

Same as the Basic, except with both arms extended over your head for the entire exercise. Raise your torso and simultaneously bring your feet to the floor and stand up, keeping arms extended over your head.

Advanced: Get-ups off Floor with Medicine Ball Overhead

Same as the Intermediate, except start by lying on the floor instead of the BOSU, with knees bent and holding a medicine ball over your head. As you begin to "get up," bring the ball down from over your head to in front of your chest.

Sets/Reps: Competitive Season—three sets of 12 to 15 reps

2. Overhead Raises with Stretch Cords or Bands

Purpose: To strengthen shoulders, back, lats, abdominals, and core.

Basic: Overhead Raises with Stretch Cords or Bands

Start by holding one end of a stretch cord in both hands and place your foot on the other end of the stretch cord on the floor to hold it in place. Give yourself enough slack so you can extend the stretch cord directly over your head, keeping your arms straight. While keeping your arms straight, raise the stretch cord directly above your shoulders and head; then, lower to start position and repeat. (See page 45.)

Intermediate: Overhead Raises with Stretch Cords or Bands in Lunge Position

Same as the Basic, except stagger your feet in a lunge position while raising the stretch cord directly over your head. Split the repetitions between each leg.

Advanced: Squat with Overhead Raises Using Kettle Bell

Start by standing with feet shoulder-width apart, holding one kettle bell with both hands. Begin by squatting back and bringing the kettle bell through your legs. Then, while extending out of the squat and returning to a standing position, simultaneously swing the kettle bell straight out in front and above your head while keeping your arms straight. Then, slowly lower the kettle bell and return to the start position. (See page 46.)

Sets/Reps: Competitive Season—three sets of 12 to 15 reps

3. Superman on BOSU

Purpose: To strengthen back, shoulders, glutes, hamstrings, abdominals, and core.

Basic: Superman on BOSU

Start by lying facedown with your hips centered on the BOSU, your legs straight and hip-width apart, and your palms facing up. Extend your shoulder blades back and down toward your spine. Inhale to prepare for the movement and then exhale as you extend your lower back, squeezing your glutes as you extend your torso up while rotating your thumbs toward the ceiling. Hold for 1 second in that position before returning to the start position. (See page 44.)

Intermediate: Superman on BOSU with Arms Overhead

Same as the Basic, except raise your arms over your head and perform the movement without rotating your thumbs toward the ceiling. (See page 44.)

Advanced: Swimming on BOSU

Start by lying facedown, balanced on your midsection over the BOSU, with legs extended and arms overhead. Raise your arms and legs off the floor, find your balance, and then perform a swimming-type movement (no need to do the crawl stroke, exactly) by fluttering your arms and legs for about 30 to 60 seconds. (See page 44.)

Sets/Reps: Competitive Season—three sets of 12 to 15 reps
Advanced: Sets/Reps: Competitive Season—three sets of 30 to 60 seconds

Distance Cyclist Program

This program includes the following exercises:

Off-Season	Preseason	Competitive Season
Fink Five	Fink Five	Fink Five
1. Ax Chop on BOSU	1. Squat, Curl, Press	1. Get-ups off BOSU
2. Dead Lifts with Dumbells	2. One-Leg Press/ Hop	2. Overhead Raises
3. Chest Flys	3. Obliques	3. Superman on BOSU
4. One-Leg Split/Squat		
5. Ab Triangles		

First Phase: Off-Season of Distance Cyclist Program

In the Off-Season, the Distance Cyclist Program starts with the Fink Five and then goes right into the following five exercises, which most practiced athletes can complete in 12 minutes. If an athlete starts with the Easy Eight warm-up routine (5 minutes), then completes the Fink Five (12 minutes), and then finishes up with the following five exercises (12 minutes), he or she can complete the entire program in less than 30 minutes.

1. Squat with Ax Chop on BOSU

Purpose: To strengthen hamstrings, quads, glutes, abdominals, arms, shoulders, and back.

Basic: Squat with Ax Chop on BOSU Using Medicine Ball

Start by standing on top of the BOSU, holding a medicine ball at shoulder height to one side with arms bent. As you are performing a squat, and at the same pace as the squat, lower the medicine ball to the opposite side across your body in a chopping motion until you complete the squat. Return to the start position, extending your legs while reversing the chopping motion, and then repeat on the same side before switching to the other side. (See page 33.)

Intermediate: Squat with Ax Chop on BOSU Using Kettle Bell

Same as the Basic, except use a kettle bell to perform the exercise.

Advanced: Side Lunge with Ax Chop on BOSU Using Kettle Bell

Start by standing on top of the BOSU, holding a kettle bell at shoulder height to one side with arms bent. As you are performing a side lunge, swing the kettle bell to the opposite side across your body in a chopping motion to the outside of your lunging leg until you complete the lunge. Return to the start position and bring the kettle bell back to the opposite shoulder by reversing the chopping motion. Repeat on the opposite side.

Sets/Reps: Off-Season—three sets of 8 to 12 reps, each side

2. Dead Lifts with Dumbbells

Purpose: To strengthen glutes, hamstrings, quads, ab/adductors, calves, and core.

Basic: Dead Lifts with Dumbbells

Start in a standing position with feet about shoulder-width apart and a dumbbell in each hand. Keep belly drawn in and shoulder blades back and down. Keeping arms straight down the entire time, lower the dumbbells toward the floor, with knees slightly bent and a straight back. Then return to a standing position by pushing through your glutes and hamstrings as you return to the start position. (See page 62.)

Intermediate: Dead Lifts with Dumbbells to Calf Raise

Same as the Basic, except as you return to start position from dead lift, go immediately onto your toes and perform a calf raise. Be sure to maintain good posture, back flat and lifting through your glutes and hamstrings. (See page 63.)

Advanced: Dead Lifts with Dumbbells to Calf Raise on One Leg

Same as the Intermediate, except you will perform the dead lift to calf raise while standing on one leg only. Be sure to maintain good posture, drawing your belly in and keeping your shoulders back and down. You can keep your off leg straight or slightly bent.

Sets/Reps: Off-Season—three sets of 8 to 12 reps

3. Chest Flys with Stretch Cords in Lunge Position

Purpose: To strengthen pectorals, shoulders, glutes, hamstrings, abdominals, core, and balance.

Basic: Chest Flys with Stretch Cords in Lunge Position

Start in a standing position, holding the ends of the stretch cord in both hands, facing away from the door/wall with your legs in a lunge position. Extend your slightly bent arms out to the sides about chest level. Inhale, then exhale as you squeeze your chest and bring your arms together in front, with palms facing down; hold, then return to the start position while keeping your arms extended from your sides. (See page 34.)

Intermediate: Chest Flys with Stretch Cords—Standing on One Leg

Same as the Basic, except start by standing on one leg. Perform the movement with the leg raised for half of the repetitions and then repeat with the other leg raised for the other half of the repetitions.

Advanced: Alternating Arm/Chest Flys with Stretch Cords—Standing on One Leg

Same as the Intermediate, except with leg raised, perform the movement with alternating arms. Start with both arms extended in front of you and then perform a fly with only one arm. Perform half of the repetitions on one leg and then switch legs and perform the remaining repetitions.

Sets/Reps: Off-Season—three sets of 8 to 12 reps

4. One-Leg Split/Squat with Elevated Leg

Purpose: To strengthen glutes, hamstrings, quads, abs, core, and balance.

Basic: One-Leg Split/Squat with Elevated Leg

Start in a standing position about 2 feet in front of a bench/chair. Bring one foot behind you and place the top of your foot on the bench/chair. Inhale, then squat down by flexing hip and knee of front leg until knee of rear leg is as close to the floor as possible. Hold, and then extend hip and knee of front leg back to start position. Repeat on that leg through a full set of repetitions and then switch legs. (See photos 32a and 32b below, but disregard kettle bell.)

Intermediate: One-Leg Split/Squat with Elevated Leg and Kettle Bell

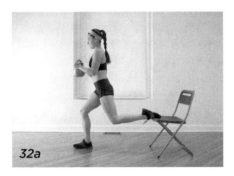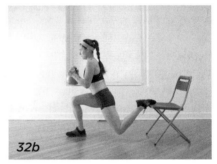

Same as the Basic, except you will perform the exercise while holding one kettle bell with both hands at your chest. (See photos 32a and 32b above.)

Advanced: One-Leg Split/Squat with Elevated Leg and Two Kettle Bells or Dumbbells

Same as the Intermediate, except hold two kettle bells or dumbbells—one in each hand at your sides—and perform the exercise.

Sets/Reps: Off-Season—three sets of 8 to 12 reps

5. Abs—Open-and-Close Triangles

Purpose: To strengthen overall core and abdominals.

Basic: Abs—Open-and-Close Triangles

Start by lying on the floor on your back with legs extended straight so they are perpendicular to the floor and your arms extended toward your knees. Your legs, torso, and arms should almost form a right triangle. Simultaneously, lower your legs together toward the floor and your arms straight over your head from your shoulders. Hold your position when you are straight but not quite touching the ground, and then return to the start position and repeat. (See page 37.)

Intermediate: Abs—Stability Ball Pass from Hands to Feet

Same as the Basic, except you start with a stability ball in your hands as you lower your arms overhead and your legs toward the floor. Then, simultaneously, raise your arms and legs together and pass the stability ball from your hands to between your feet and repeat the movement. Continue passing the ball from your hands to your feet at each return to starting point and make the movement continuous. (See page 38.)

Advanced: Stability Ball Pass from Hands to Feet with Raised Torso

Same as the Intermediate, except raise your torso off the floor every time you raise your arms back to the straight position, with or without the stability ball.

Sets/Reps: Off-Season—three sets of 8 to 12 reps

Second Phase: Preseason Distance Cyclist Program (reps increase to 10–12 range)

Once we are about eight to twelve weeks away from our first major race of the year, we will transition into the Preseason Phase of the Distance Cyclist Program. This phase starts with the Fink Five and then goes right into the following three exercises, which most practiced athletes can complete in about 7.5 minutes. If an athlete starts with the Easy Eight warm-up routine (5 minutes), then completes the Fink Five (12 minutes), and then finishes up with the following three Preseason Exercises (7.5 minutes), he or she can complete the entire Preseason Program in less than 25 minutes.

1. Squat to Curl and Press

Purpose: To strengthen glutes, hamstrings, biceps, shoulders, and core.

Basic: Squat to Curl and Press

Start in a standing position with a dumbbell in each hand. Begin by inhaling, and then perform a freestanding squat. As you return from the squat position, begin to curl the dumbbells as you get to the start position and then press the dumbbells over your head. Return the dumbbells to your sides and repeat. (See page 75.)

Intermediate: Squat on BOSU, Curl and Press

Same as the Basic, except start by standing on the BOSU.

Advanced: Squat on One Leg, Curl and Press

Same as the Basic, except start by raising one leg straight up, with knee bent and parallel to the ground. Swing leg back, perform squat with other leg, then curl and press the weights over your head, and then return the weights to your sides. Repeat with same leg through a complete set of repetitions before switching to the other leg.

Sets/Reps: Preseason—three sets of 10 to 12 reps

2. One-Leg Press to Hop (with or without dumbbells)

Purpose: To strengthen glutes, hamstrings, quads, ankles, core, and balance, and to develop power.

Basic: One-Leg Press with Foot on Step (with or without dumbbells)

Start by standing in a lunge position with one foot on the step and the other foot behind, with knee bent almost to the floor. Perform a one-leg press with the leg on the step, and rise to a standing position while bringing the opposite leg up with raised knee. Return to the start position and repeat on that leg and then switch to the other leg. (See page 40.)

Intermediate: One-Leg Press to Hop with Foot on Step (with or without dumbbells)

Same as the Basic, except after you complete the press, hop on the same leg while keeping the opposite leg raised in a chair pose. Return to the start position and repeat on the same leg before switching to the opposite leg for the remaining repetitions. (See page 41.)

Advanced: One-Leg Press to Hop with Foot on BOSU (with or without dumbbells)

Same as the Intermediate, except start with one foot on the BOSU. Then, after you complete the press, hop on that same leg while raising the opposite knee in a chair pose. Repeat on the same leg before switching to the opposite leg.

Sets/Reps: Preseason—three sets of 10 to 12 reps, each leg

3. Obliques over BOSU

Purpose: To strengthen obliques and core.

Basic: Obliques over BOSU

Start by lying on the BOSU with the small of your back centered on top, both arms behind your head, and your feet on the floor. Slightly raise your torso off the BOSU while pointing one elbow toward the opposite knee. Hold and return to the start position and then repeat with the opposite elbow toward the other knee. Repeat by alternating sides. (See page 51.)

Intermediate: Obliques over BOSU with One Leg Raised

Same as the Basic, except with both hands behind your head, slightly raise your torso while raising the left leg and pointing the right elbow toward the left knee. Outstretched leg should remain off the floor. Repeat on that side and then switch legs and repeat on the other side. (See page 52.)

Advanced: Bicycles over BOSU with Legs Raised

Same as the Intermediate, except with both hands behind your head, raise your torso and legs off the floor so you are balanced on the BOSU. Extend one leg straight and keep the other leg bent. Start the movement by bringing the knee of the extended leg to the opposite elbow so they make contact. Repeat this movement with the opposite arm and leg, alternating the movement from one side to the other while maintaining balance on the BOSU. (See page 52.)

Sets/Reps: Preseason—three sets of 10 to 12 reps, each side

Third Phase: Competitive Season of Distance Cyclist Program (reps increase to 12–15 range)

Once we have completed our first major race of the year, we will transition into the Competitive-Season Phase of the Distance Cyclist Program. This phase starts with the Fink Five and then goes right into the following three exercises, which most practiced athletes can complete in about 7.5 minutes. If an athlete starts with the Easy Eight warm-up routine (5 minutes), then completes the Fink Five (12 minutes), and then finishes up with the following three Competitive-Season Exercises (7.5 minutes), he or she can complete the entire Competitive-Season Program in less than 25 minutes. Additional Note: As part of a proper pre-race taper, it is our general suggestion not to perform strength training during the week immediately preceding a major race.

1. Get-ups off BOSU with Arms at Your Sides

Purpose: To strengthen core and abdominals, glutes, quads, core, and hamstrings.

Basic: Get-ups off the BOSU with Arms at Your Sides

Start by sitting on the BOSU with arms at your sides and bent knees. Extend your torso back so you are completely parallel to the floor and legs are raised off the floor. Then, raise torso and simultaneously put your feet on the floor and stand straight up. Then, return to the start position and repeat. (See page 41.)

Intermediate: Get-ups off BOSU with Arms Raised

Same as the Basic, except with both arms extended over your head for the entire exercise. Raise your torso and simultaneously bring your feet to the floor and stand up, keeping arms extended over your head.

Advanced: Get-ups off Floor with Medicine Ball Overhead

Same as the Intermediate, except start by lying on the floor instead of the BOSU, with knees bent and holding a medicine ball over your head. As you begin to "get up," bring the ball down from over your head to in front of your chest.

Sets/Reps: Competitive Season—three sets of 12 to 15 reps

2. Overhead Raises with Stretch Cords or Bands

Purpose: To strengthen shoulders, back, lats, abdominals, and core.

Basic: Overhead Raises with Stretch Cords or Bands

Start by holding one end of a stretch cord in both hands and place your foot on the other end of the stretch cord on the floor to hold it in place. Give yourself enough slack so you can extend the stretch cord directly over your head, keeping your arms straight. While keeping your arms straight, raise the stretch cord directly above your shoulders and head; then, lower to start position and repeat.

Intermediate: Overhead Raises with Stretch Cords or Bands in Lunge Position

Same as the Basic, except stagger your feet in a lunge position while raising the stretch cord directly over your head. Split the repetitions between each leg. (See page 45.)

Advanced: Squat with Overhead Raises Using Kettle Bell

Start by standing with feet shoulder-width apart, holding one kettle bell with both hands. Begin by squatting back and bringing the kettle bell through

your legs. Then, while extending out of the squat and returning to a standing position, simultaneously swing the kettle bell straight out in front and above your head while keeping your arms straight. Then, slowly lower the kettle bell and return to the start position. (See page 46.)

Sets/Reps: Competitive Season—three sets of 12 to 15 reps

3. Superman on BOSU

Purpose: To strengthen back, shoulders, glutes, hamstrings, abdominals, and core.

Basic: Superman on BOSU

Start by lying facedown with your hips centered on the BOSU, your legs straight and hip-width apart, and your palms facing up. Extend your shoulder blades back and down toward your spine. Inhale to prepare for the movement and then exhale as you extend your lower back, squeezing your glutes as you extend your torso up while rotating your thumbs toward the ceiling. Hold for 1 second in that position before returning to the start position. (See page 44.)

Intermediate: Superman on BOSU with Arms Overhead

Same as the Basic, except raise your arms over your head and perform the movement without rotating your thumbs toward the ceiling. (See page 44.)

Advanced: Swimming on BOSU

Start by lying facedown, balanced on your midsection over the BOSU, with legs extended and arms overhead. Raise your arms and legs off the floor, find your balance, and then perform a swimming-type movement (no need to do the crawl stroke, exactly) by fluttering your arms and legs for about 30 to 60 seconds. (See page 44.)

Sets/Reps: Competitive Season—three sets of 12 to 15 reps
Advanced: Sets/Reps: Competitive Season—three sets of 30 to 60 seconds

Swimmers—Distance and Open-Water Program

This program includes the following exercises:

Off-Season	Preseason	Competitive Season
Fink Five	Fink Five	Fink Five
1. Ax Chop on BOSU	1. Squat, Curl, Press	1. Get-ups off BOSU
2. Pullovers	2. Overhead Raises	2. One-Leg Squat with
3. Jump Squats	3. Superman on BOSU	DB Rotation
4. Side Lunge with		3. Side Planks
Front Raise		
5. Rear Delt Flys		

First Phase: Off-Season of Swimmers—Distance and Open-Water Program

In the Off-Season, the Swimmers—Distance and Open-Water Program starts with the Fink Five and then goes right into the following five exercises, which most practiced athletes can complete in 12 minutes. If an athlete starts with the Easy Eight warm-up routine (5 minutes), then completes the Fink Five (12 minutes), and then finishes up with the following five exercises (12 minutes), he or she can complete the entire program in less than 30 minutes.

1. Squat with Ax Chop on BOSU

Purpose: To strengthen hamstrings, quads, glutes, abdominals, arms, shoulders, and back.

Basic: Squat with Ax Chop on BOSU Using Medicine Ball

Start by standing on top of the BOSU, holding a medicine ball at shoulder height to one side with arms bent. As you are performing a squat, and at the same pace as the squat, lower the medicine ball to the opposite side across your body in a chopping motion until you complete the squat. Return to the start position, extending the legs while reversing the chopping motion, and then repeat on the same side before switching to the other side. (See page 33.)

Intermediate: Squat with Ax Chop on BOSU Using Kettle Bell

Same as the Basic, except use a kettle bell to perform the exercise.

Advanced: Side Lunge with Ax Chop on BOSU Using Kettle Bell

Start by standing on top of the BOSU, holding a kettle bell at shoulder height to one side with arms bent. As you are performing a side lunge, swing the kettle bell to the opposite side across your body in a chopping motion to the outside of your lunging leg until you complete the lunge. Return to the start position and bring the kettle bell back to the opposite shoulder by reversing the chopping motion. Repeat on the opposite side.

Sets/Reps: Off-Season—three sets of 8 to 12 reps, each side

2. Pullovers with Hip Extension on Stability Ball with Medicine Ball

Purpose: To strengthen lats, pectorals, glutes, hamstrings, and core.

Basic: Pullovers with Hip Extension on Stability Ball Using a Medicine Ball

Start by lying on the stability ball with your back, neck, and head resting on top of the ball and your hips extended and knees bent, keeping quadriceps parallel to the floor. Raise the medicine ball with arms straight above your chest, inhale, and keep hips and knees in a straight line as you extend the medicine ball over your head, bringing your arms as close to parallel to the floor as possible. Hold that position for 1 second, and then while exhaling, raise the ball back to the start position and repeat. (See page 43.)

Intermediate: Pullovers on Stability Ball with Dumbbells

Same as the Basic, except that you use a dumbbell in each hand and perform the same movement with elbows slightly bent.

Advanced: Pullovers on Stability Ball with Medicine Ball and One Leg Raised

Same as the Basic, except you perform the exercise with one leg raised.

Sets/Reps: Off-Season—three sets of 8 to 12 reps

3. Jump Squats onto Step or Box

Purpose: To strengthen glutes, hamstrings, quads, ankles, abs, core, and balance.

Basic: Jump Squats onto Step or Box

Start in a standing position with your feet about shoulder-width apart in front of a step or box. With your arms at your sides, inhale and perform a deep squat. From the deep squat position, exhale and jump onto the step or box with both feet and land in a squat position. Step off step or box and repeat the squat and jump. (See page 50.)

Intermediate: Jump Squats onto BOSU

Same as the Basic, except you will start by standing in front of a BOSU, jumping onto it, and landing in a squat position. Step off the BOSU and perform the squat and jump again.

Advanced: Jump Squats on the BOSU

Start by standing on the BOSU. Perform a deep squat and jump by extending your legs, hips, and glutes straight up, and then landing in a deep squat position back on the BOSU. Repeat the jump and squat.

Sets/Reps: Off-Season—three sets of 8 to 12 reps

4. Side Lunge with Front Raise

Purpose: To strengthen glutes, hamstrings, quads, ab/adductors, shoulders, and core.

Basic: Side Lunge with Front Raise

Start in a standing position with a dumbbell in each hand at your sides. Perform a side lunge, keeping your hips back and lunging leg bent while your other leg stays straight. From that position raise your arms with dumbbells out straight to shoulder height, hold, and then simultaneously bring your arms back to your sides while extending your hips, glutes, and quads back to the start position. Perform half of the repetitions on one leg and then switch and perform half of the repetitions on the other leg. (See page 35.)

Intermediate: Side Lunge onto Step with Front Raise

Same as the Basic, except side-lunge onto a step.

Advanced: Side Lunge onto BOSU with One-Arm Front Raise

Same as the Intermediate, except side-lunge onto a BOSU so your foot strikes the center of the BOSU and raise the same side arm. Then, repeat with other leg and arm.

Sets/Reps: Off-Season—three sets of 8 to 12 reps / Advanced—three sets of 8 to 12 reps, each side

5. Rear Deltoid Flys in Stork Position

Purpose: To strengthen deltoids, rhomboids, hamstrings, quads, core, and balance.

Basic: Rear Deltoid Flys in Stork Position

Start in a standing position with a dumbbell in each hand. Raise one leg straight behind you and balance on the other leg in a stork position, letting your arms hang straight down. Depress your shoulder blades toward your spine and raise the dumbbells with slightly bent arms out to the sides, but not higher than shoulder height. Hold for a 2-second count and then return arms back to the start position and repeat. Keep hands soft as you squeeze your shoulder blades together to elevate the weights. Perform half the repetitions on one leg and then switch and perform half the repetitions on the other leg. (See page 36.)

Intermediate: Rear Deltoid Flys in Stork Position, Alternating Arms

Same as the Basic, except perform this exercise by raising one arm at a time and alternating arms. Perform half of the repetitions on one leg and then switch and perform half of the repetitions on the other leg.

Advanced: Rear Deltoid Flys with One-Leg Squat in Stork Position

Same as the Basic, except start this exercise from the stork position and begin with a one-leg squat; then, as you extend from the squat, simultaneously raise the weights as you return to the start position. Perform half of the repetitions on one leg and then switch and perform half of the repetitions on the other leg.

Sets/Reps: Off-Season—three sets of 8 to 12 reps

Second Phase: Swimmers—Distance and Open-Water Program (reps increase to 10–12 range)

Once we are about eight to twelve weeks away from our first major race of the year, we will transition into the Preseason Phase of the Swimmers—Distance and Open-Water Program. This phase starts with the Fink Five and then goes right into the following three exercises, which most practiced athletes can complete in about 7.5 minutes. If an athlete starts with the Easy Eight warm-up routine (5 minutes), then completes the Fink Five (12 minutes), and then finishes up with the following three Preseason Exercises (7.5 minutes), he or she can complete the entire Preseason Program in less than 25 minutes.

1. Squat to Curl and Press

Purpose: To strengthen glutes, hamstrings, biceps, shoulders, and core.

Basic: Squat to Curl and Press

Start in a standing position with a dumbbell in each hand. Begin by inhaling, and then perform a freestanding squat. As you return from the squat position, begin to curl the dumbbells as you get to the start position and then press the dumbbells over your head. Return the dumbbells to your sides and repeat. (See page 75.)

Intermediate: Squat on BOSU, Curl and Press

Same as the Basic, except start by standing on the BOSU.

Advanced: Squat on One Leg, Curl and Press

Same as the Basic, except start by raising one leg straight up, with knee bent and parallel to the ground. Swing leg back, perform squat with other leg, then curl and press the weights over your head, and then return the weights to your sides. Repeat with same leg through a complete set of repetitions before switching to the other leg.

Sets/Reps: Preseason—three sets of 10 to 12 reps

2. Overhead Raises with Stretch Cords or Bands

Purpose: To strengthen shoulders, back, lats, abdominals, and core.

Basic: Overhead Raises with Stretch Cords or Bands

Start by holding one end of a stretch cord in both hands and place your foot on the other end of the stretch cord on the floor to hold it in place. Give yourself enough slack so you can extend the stretch cord directly over your head, keeping your arms straight. While keeping your arms straight, raise the stretch cord directly above your shoulders and head; then, lower to start position and repeat.

Intermediate: Overhead Raises with Stretch Cords or Bands in Lunge Position

Same as the Basic, except stagger your feet in a lunge position while raising the stretch cord directly over your head. Split the repetitions between each leg. (See page 45.)

Advanced: Squat with Overhead Raises Using Kettle Bell

Start by standing with feet shoulder-width apart, holding one kettle bell with both hands. Begin by squatting back and bringing the kettle bell through your legs. Then, while extending out of the squat and returning to a standing position, simultaneously swing the kettle bell straight out in front and above your head while keeping your arms straight. Then, slowly lower the kettle bell and return to the start position. (See page 46.)

Sets/Reps: Preseason—three sets of 10 to 12 reps, each leg /
Advanced—three sets of 10 to 12 reps

3. Superman on BOSU

Purpose: To strengthen back, shoulders, glutes, hamstrings, abdominals, and core.

Basic: Superman on BOSU

Start by lying facedown with your hips centered on the BOSU, your legs straight and hip-width apart, and your palms facing up. Extend your shoulder blades back and down toward your spine. Inhale to prepare for the movement and then exhale as you extend your lower back, squeezing your glutes as you extend your torso up while rotating your thumbs toward the ceiling. Hold for 1 second in that position before returning to the start position. (See page 44.)

Intermediate: Superman on BOSU with Arms Overhead

Same as the Basic, except raise your arms over your head and perform the movement without rotating your thumbs toward the ceiling. (See page 44.)

Advanced: Swimming on BOSU

Start by lying facedown, balanced on your midsection over the BOSU, with legs extended and arms overhead. Raise your arms and legs off the floor, find your balance, and then perform a swimming-type movement (no need to do the crawl stroke, exactly) by fluttering your arms and legs for about 30 to 60 seconds. (See page 44.)

Sets/Reps: Preseason—three sets of 10 to 12 reps
Advanced: Sets/Reps: Preseason—three sets of 30 to 60 seconds

Third Phase: Competitive Season of Swimmers—Distance and Open-Water Program (reps increase to 15–20 range)

Once we have completed our first major race of the year, we will transition into the Competitive-Season Phase of the Swimmers—Distance and Open-Water Program. This phase starts with the Fink Five and then goes right into the following three exercises, which most practiced athletes can complete in about 7.5 minutes. If an athlete starts with the Easy Eight warm-up routine

(5 minutes), then completes the Fink Five (12 minutes), and then finishes up with the following three Competitive-Season Exercises (7.5 minutes), he or she can complete the entire Competitive-Season Program in less than 25 minutes. Additional Note: As part of a proper pre-race taper, it is our general suggestion not to perform strength training during the week immediately preceding a major race.

1. Get-ups off BOSU with Arms at Your Sides

Purpose: To strengthen core and abdominals, glutes, quads, and hamstrings.

Basic: Get-ups off the BOSU with Arms at Your Sides

Start by sitting on the BOSU with arms at your sides and bent knees. Extend your torso back so you are completely parallel to the floor and legs are raised off the floor. Then, raise torso and simultaneously put your feet on the floor and stand straight up. Then, return to the start position and repeat. (See page 41.)

Intermediate: Get-ups off BOSU with Arms Raised

Same as the Basic, except with both arms extended over your head for the entire exercise. Raise your torso and simultaneously bring your feet to the floor and stand up, keeping arms extended over your head.

Advanced: Get-ups off Floor with Medicine Ball Overhead

Same as the Intermediate, except start by lying on the floor instead of the BOSU, with knees bent and holding a medicine ball over your head. As you begin to "get up," bring the ball down from over your head to in front of your chest.

Sets/Reps: Competitive Season—three sets of 12 to 15 reps

2. One-Leg Squats with Dumbbell Reach and Rotation

Purpose: To strengthen ab/adductors, glutes, hamstrings, quadriceps, hip flexors, shoulders, core, and obliques.

Basic: One-Leg Squats with Dumbbell Reach and Rotation

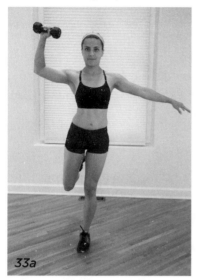
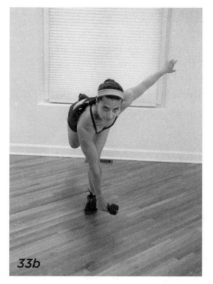

33a 33b

Start by standing on one leg with knee slightly bent. Your opposite arm is raised with bent elbow at shoulder height and a dumbbell in your hand. Simultaneously, perform a one-leg squat by flexing at your hip and knee as you reach the dumbbell across your body toward the outside of the opposite foot. From the squat position, extend hip and knee and raise dumbbell back across body and externally rotate arm while keeping your elbow bent and bringing it back to the start position. (See photos 33a and 33b above.) Note: There are no progressions for this exercise.

Sets/Reps: Competitive Season—three sets of 12 to 15 reps, each leg

3. Side Planks

Purpose: To strengthen obliques, abdominals, core, and shoulders.

Basic: Side Plank on Floor

Start by lying on your side on the floor with your upper body resting on your bent elbow under your shoulder and your other arm at your side. Draw in your belly and hold, while raising your hip and torso off the floor with weight on your forearm until there is a straight line from your ankles to your head.

Hold for 5- to 10-second count and maintain drawn-in belly as you lower hips to the floor. Repeat on your other side. (See page 76.)

Intermediate: Side Plank on Floor with Arm Raise

Same as the Basic, except raise and lower your top arm repeatedly with palm facing up while holding the position for a 15- to 30-second count; then, repeat on your other side.

Advanced: Side Plank on Floor with Ab Crunch

Same as the Basic, except place the hand of your top arm behind your head with bent elbow. While holding plank position, rotate your elbow toward the floor and repeat for the desired number of repetitions, and then repeat on your other side. (See page 77.)

Sets/Reps: Competitive Season—three sets of 12 to 15 reps, each side

Cross-Country Skier Program

This program includes the following exercises:

Off-Season	Preseason	Competitive Season
Fink Five	Fink Five	Fink Five
1. Ax Chop on BOSU	1. Side Lunge with	1. Get-ups off BOSU
2. Chest Flys	Front Raise	2. Overhead Raises
3. One-Leg Split/	2. One-Leg Press/Hop	3. Superman on BOSU
Squat	3. Obliques	
4. Rear Delt Flys		
5. Sliders to the Side		

First Phase: Off-Season of Cross-Country Skier Program

In the Off-Season, the Cross-Country Skier Program starts with the Fink Five and then goes right into the following five exercises, which most practiced athletes can complete in 12 minutes. If an athlete starts with the Easy Eight warm-up routine (5 minutes), then completes the Fink Five (12 minutes), and then finishes up with the following five exercises (12 minutes), he or she can complete the entire program in less than 30 minutes.

1. Squat with Ax Chop on BOSU

Purpose: To strengthen hamstrings, quads, glutes, abdominals, arms, shoulders, core, and back.

Basic: Squat with Ax Chop on BOSU using Medicine Ball

Start by standing on top of the BOSU, holding a medicine ball at shoulder height to one side, with arms bent. As you are performing a squat, and at the same pace as the squat, lower the medicine ball to the opposite side across your body in a chopping motion until you complete the squat. Return to the start position, extending the legs while reversing the chopping motion, and then repeat on the same side before switching to the other side. (See page 33.)

Intermediate: Squat with Ax Chop on BOSU Using Kettle Bell

Same as the Basic, except use a kettle bell to perform the exercise.

Advanced: Side Lunge with Ax Chop on BOSU Using Kettle Bell

Start by standing on top of the BOSU, holding a kettle bell at shoulder height to one side, with arms bent. As you are performing a side lunge, swing the kettle bell to the opposite side across your body in a chopping motion to the outside of your lunging leg until you complete the lunge. Return to the start position and bring the kettle bell back to the opposite shoulder by reversing the chopping motion. Repeat on the opposite side.

Sets/Reps: Off-Season—three sets of 8 to 12 reps, each side

2. Chest Flys with Stretch Cords in Lunge Position

Purpose: To strengthen pectorals, shoulders, glutes, hamstrings, abdominals, core, and balance.

Basic: Chest Flys with Stretch Cords in Lunge Position

Start in a standing position, holding the ends of the stretch cord in both hands facing away from the door/wall with your legs in a lunge position. Extend your slightly bent arms out to the sides about chest level. Inhale, then exhale as you squeeze your chest and bring your arms together in front with palms facing down; hold, then return to the start position while keeping your arms extended from your sides. (See page 34.)

Intermediate: Chest Flys with Stretch Cords, Standing on One Leg

Same as the Basic, except start by standing on one leg. Perform the movement with one leg raised for half of the repetitions, and then repeat with the other leg raised for the other half of the repetitions.

Advanced: Alternating Arm/Chest Flys with Stretch Cords, Standing on One Leg

Same as the Intermediate, except with leg raised, perform the movement with alternating arms. Start with both arms extended in front of you and then perform a fly with only one arm. Perform half of the repetitions on one leg and then switch legs and perform the remaining repetitions.

Sets/Reps: Off-Season—three sets of 8 to 12 reps

3. One-Leg Split/Squat with Elevated Leg

Purpose: To strengthen glutes, hamstrings, quads, abs, core, and balance.

Basic: One-Leg Split/Squat with Elevated Leg

Start in a standing position about 2 feet in front of a bench/chair. Bring one foot behind you and place the top of your foot on the bench/chair. Inhale, then squat down by flexing the hip and knee of front leg until knee of rear leg is as close to the floor as possible. Hold, and then extend hip and knee of front leg back to start position. Repeat on that leg through a full set of repetitions and then switch legs. (See page 84, but disregard kettle bell.)

Intermediate: One-Leg Split/Squat with Elevated Leg and Kettle Bell

Same as the Basic, except you will perform the exercise while holding one kettle bell with both hands at your chest. (See page 84.)

Advanced: One-Leg Split/Squat with Elevated Leg and Two Kettle Bells or Dumbbells

Same as the Intermediate, except hold two kettle bells or dumbbells—one in each hand—and perform the exercise.

Sets/Reps: Off-Season—three sets of 8 to 12 reps

4. Rear Deltoid Flys in Stork Position

Purpose: To strengthen deltoids, rhomboids, hamstrings, quads, core, and balance.

Basic: Rear Deltoid Flys in Stork Position

Start in a standing position with a dumbbell in each hand. Raise one leg straight behind you and balance on the other leg in a stork position, letting your arms hang straight down. Depress your shoulder blades toward your spine and raise the dumbbells with slightly bent arms out to the sides, but not higher than shoulder height. Hold for a 2-second count and then return arms back to the start position and repeat. Keep hands soft as you squeeze your shoulder blades together to elevate the weights. Perform half the repetitions on one leg and then switch and perform half the repetitions on the other leg. (See page 36.)

Intermediate: Rear Deltoid Flys in Stork Position, Alternating Arms

Same as the Basic, except perform this exercise by raising one arm at a time and alternating arms. Perform half of the repetitions on one leg and then switch and perform half of the repetitions on the other leg.

Advanced: Rear Deltoid Flys with One-Leg Squat in Stork Position

Same as the Basic, except start this exercise from the stork position and begin with a one-leg squat; then, as you extend from the squat, simultaneously raise the weights as you return to the start position. Perform half of the repetitions on one leg and then switch and perform half of the repetitions on the other leg.

Sets/Reps: Off-Season—three sets of 8 to 12 reps

5. Sliders to Side

Purpose: To strengthen ab/adductors, glutes, hamstrings, quads, abs, core, and balance.

Basic: Sliders to the Side

This exercise is best performed on a hardwood floor or other semi-slick surface. Start in a standing position with a piece of paper under one foot. Begin by sliding the foot with the paper under it to the side, keeping the leg straight as you bend the opposite hip and knee into a lunge position. Use your glutes and hamstrings to return your leg next to the other leg in a standing position. Repeat with that leg through a full set of repetitions and then repeat with paper under the other foot. (See photos 34a and 34b, next page.)

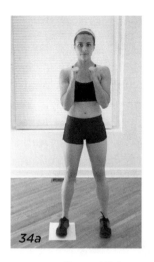
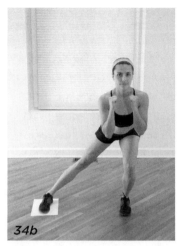

Intermediate: Sliders to Side (with dumbbells)

Same as the Basic, except hold a dumbbell in each hand while performing the movement.

Advanced: Sliders to Half-Circle (with or without dumbbells)

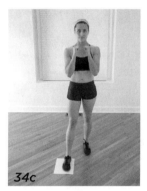
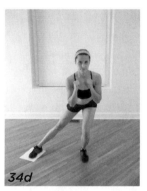
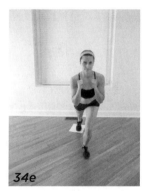

Start in staggered-stance position with a piece of paper under the foot in front (starting at twelve o'clock). Begin by sliding the front foot around in a half-circle all the way to the six o'clock position while bending at the hip and knee on the other leg. Repeat on that leg through a full set of repetitions and then repeat with paper under the other foot. To add difficulty, hold a dumb-bell in each hand. (See photos 34c, 34d, and 34e above.)

Sets/Reps: Off-Season—three sets of 8 to 12 reps, each leg

Second Phase: Cross-Country Skier Program (reps increase to 10–12 range)

Once we are about eight to twelve weeks away from our first major race of the year, we will transition into the Preseason Phase of the Cross-Country Skier Program. This phase starts with the Fink Five and then goes right into the following three exercises, which most practiced athletes can complete in about 7.5 minutes. Therefore, in an athlete starts with the Easy Eight warm-up routine (5 minutes), then completes the Fink Five (12 minutes), and then finishes up with the following three Preseason Exercises (7.5 minutes), he or she can complete the entire Preseason Program in less than 25 minutes.

1. Side Lunge with Front Raise

Purpose: To strengthen glutes, hamstrings, quads, ab/adductors, shoulders, and core.

Basic: Side Lunge with Front Raise

Start in a standing position with a dumbbell in each hand at your sides. Perform a side lunge, keeping your hips back and lunging leg bent while your other leg stays straight. From that position raise your arms with dumbbells out straight to shoulder height, hold, and then simultaneously bring your arms back to your sides while extending your hips, glutes, and quads back to the start position. Perform half of the repetitions on one leg and then switch and perform half of the repetitions on the other leg. (See page 35.)

Intermediate: Side Lunge onto Step with Front Raise

Same as the Basic, except side-lunge onto a step.

Advanced: Side Lunge onto BOSU with One-Arm Front Raise

Same as the Intermediate, except side-lunge onto a BOSU so your foot strikes the center of it, and raise the same side arm. Then, repeat with other leg and arm.

Sets/Reps: Preseason—three sets of 10 to 12 reps / Advanced—three sets of 10 to 12 reps, each side

2. One-Leg Press to Hop (with or without dumbbells)

Purpose: To strengthen glutes, hamstrings, quads, ankles, core, and balance, and to develop power.

Basic: One-Leg Press with Foot on Step (with or without dumbbells)

Start by standing in a lunge position with one foot on the step and the other foot behind, with knee bent almost to the floor. Perform a one-leg press with the leg on the step, and rise to a standing position while bringing the opposite leg up with raised knee. Return to the start position and repeat on that leg and then switch to the other leg. (See page 40.)

Intermediate: One-Leg Press to Hop with Foot on Step (with or without dumbbells)

Same as the Basic, except after you complete the press, hop on the same leg while keeping the opposite leg raised in a chair pose. Return to the start position and repeat on the same leg before switching to the opposite leg for the remaining repetitions. (See page 41.)

Advanced: One-Leg Press to Hop with Foot on BOSU (with or without dumbbells)

Same as the Intermediate, except start with one foot on the BOSU. Then, after you complete the press, hop on that same leg while raising the opposite knee in a chair pose. Repeat on the same leg before switching to the opposite leg.

Sets/Reps: Preseason—three sets of 10 to 12 reps, each leg

3. Obliques over BOSU

Purpose: To strengthen obliques and core.

Basic: Obliques over BOSU

Start by lying on the BOSU with the small of your back centered on top, both arms behind your head, and your feet on the floor. Slightly raise your torso off the BOSU while pointing one elbow toward the opposite knee. Hold and return to the start position and then repeat with the opposite elbow toward the other knee. Repeat by alternating sides. (See page 51.)

Intermediate: Obliques over BOSU with One Leg Raised

Same as the Basic, except with both hands behind your head, slightly raise your torso while raising the left leg and pointing the right elbow toward the left knee. Outstretched leg should remain off the floor. Repeat on that side and then switch legs and repeat on the other side. (See page 52.)

Advanced: Bicycles over BOSU with Legs Raised

Same as the Intermediate, except with both hands behind your head, raise your torso and legs off the floor so you are balanced on the BOSU. Extend one leg straight and keep the other leg bent. Start the movement by bringing the knee of the extended leg to the opposite elbow so they make contact. Repeat this movement with the opposite arm and leg, alternating the movement from one side to the other while maintaining balance on the BOSU. (See page 52.)

Sets/Reps: Preseason—three sets of 10 to 12 reps, each side

Third Phase: Competitive Season of Cross-Country Skier Program (reps increase to 12–15 range)

Once we have completed our first major race of the year, we will transition into the Competitive-Season Phase of the Cross-Country Skier Program. This phase starts with the Fink Five and then goes right into the following three exercises, which most practiced athletes can complete in about 7.5 minutes. If an athlete starts with the Easy Eight warm-up routine (5 minutes), then completes the Fink Five (12 minutes), and then finishes up with the following three Competitive-Season Exercises (7.5 minutes), he or she can complete the entire Competitive-Season Program in less than 25 minutes. Additional Note: As part of a proper pre-race taper, it is our general suggestion not to perform strength training during the week immediately preceding a major race.

1. Get-ups off BOSU with Arms at Your Sides

Purpose: To strengthen core and abdominals, glutes, quads, core, and hamstrings.

Basic: Get-ups off the BOSU with Arms at Your Sides

Start by sitting on the BOSU with arms at your sides and bent knees. Extend your torso back so you are completely parallel to the floor and legs are raised off the floor. Then, raise torso and simultaneously put your feet on the floor and stand straight up. Then, return to the start position and repeat. (See page 41.)

Intermediate: Get-ups off BOSU with Arms Raised

Same as the Basic, except with both arms extended over your head for the entire exercise. Raise your torso and simultaneously bring your feet to the floor and stand up, keeping arms extended over your head.

Advanced: Get-ups off Floor with Medicine Ball Overhead

Same as the Intermediate, except start by lying on the floor instead of the BOSU, with knees bent and holding a medicine ball over your head. As you begin to "get up," bring the ball down from over your head to in front of your chest.

Sets/Reps: Competitive Season—three sets of 12 to 15 reps

2. Overhead Raises with Stretch Cords or Bands

Purpose: To strengthen shoulders, back, lats, abdominals, and core.

Basic: Overhead Raises with Stretch Cords or Bands

Start by holding one end of a stretch cord in both hands and place your foot on the other end of the stretch cord on the floor to hold it in place. Give yourself enough slack so you can extend the stretch cord directly over your head, keeping your arms straight. While keeping your arms straight, raise the stretch cord directly above your shoulders and head; then, lower to start position and repeat.

Intermediate: Overhead Raises with Stretch Cords or Bands in Lunge Position

Same as the Basic, except stagger your feet in a lunge position while raising the stretch cord directly over your head. Split the repetitions between each leg. (See page 45.)

Advanced: Squat with Overhead Raises Using Kettle Bell

Start by standing with feet shoulder-width apart, holding one kettle bell with both hands. Begin by squatting back and bringing the kettle bell through your legs. Then, while extending out of the squat and returning to a standing position, simultaneously swing the kettle bell straight out in front and above your head while keeping your arms straight. Then, slowly lower the kettle bell and return to the start position. (See page 46.)

Sets/Reps: Competitive Season—three sets of 12 to 15 reps

3. Superman on BOSU

Purpose: To strengthen back, shoulders, glutes, hamstrings, abdominals, and core.

Basic: Superman on BOSU

Start by lying facedown with your hips centered on the BOSU, your legs straight and hip-width apart, and your palms facing up. Extend your shoulder blades back and down toward your spine. Inhale to prepare for the movement and then exhale as you extend your lower back, squeezing your glutes as you extend your torso up while rotating your thumbs toward the ceiling. Hold for 1 second in that position before returning to the start position. (See page 44.)

Intermediate: Superman on BOSU with Arms Overhead

Same as the Basic, except raise your arms over your head and perform the movement without rotating your thumbs toward ceiling. (See page 44.)

Advanced: Swimming on BOSU

Start by lying facedown, balanced on your midsection over the BOSU, with legs extended and arms overhead. Raise your arms and legs off the floor, find your balance, and then perform a swimming-type movement (no need to do the crawl stroke, exactly) by fluttering your arms and legs for about 30 to 60 seconds. (See page 44.)

Sets/Reps: Competitive Season—three sets of 12 to 15 reps
Advanced: Sets/Reps: Competitive Season—three sets of 30 to 60 seconds

Duathlete Program

This program includes the following exercises:

Off-Season	Preseason	Competitive Season
Fink Five	Fink Five	Fink Five
1. Ax Chop on BOSU	1. Lateral Lunge	1. Rear Delt Flys
2. Dumbbell Arm Swings	2. One-Leg Press/Hop	2. Superman on BOSU
3. Jump Squats	3. Get-ups off BOSU	3. Overhead Raises
4. Side Lunge with Front Raise		
5. Obliques		

First Phase: Off-Season of Duathlete Program

In the Off-Season, the Duathlete Program starts with the Fink Five and then goes right into the following five exercises, which most practiced athletes can complete in 12 minutes. If an athlete starts with the Easy Eight warm-up routine (5 minutes), then completes the Fink Five (12 minutes), and then finishes up with the following five exercises (12 minutes), he or she can complete the entire program in less then 30 minutes.

1. Squat with Ax Chop on BOSU

Purpose: To strengthen hamstrings, quads, glutes, abdominals, arms, shoulders, and back.

Basic: Squat with Ax Chop on BOSU Using Medicine Ball

Start by standing on top of the BOSU and holding a medicine ball at shoulder height to one side, with arms bent. As you are performing a squat, and at the same pace as the squat, lower the medicine ball to the opposite side across your body in a chopping motion until you complete the squat. Return to the start position, extending the legs while reversing the chopping motion, and then repeat on the same side before switching to the other side. (See page 33.)

Intermediate: Squat with Ax Chop on BOSU Using Kettle Bell

Same as the Basic, except use a kettle bell to perform the exercise.

Advanced: Side Lunge with Ax Chop on BOSU Using Kettle Bell

Start by standing on top of the BOSU and holding a kettle bell at shoulder height to one side, with arms bent. As you are performing a side lunge, swing the kettle bell to the opposite side across your body in a chopping motion to the outside of your lunging leg until you complete the lunge. Return to the start position and bring the kettle bell back to the opposite shoulder by reversing the chopping motion. Repeat on the opposite side.

Sets/Reps: Off-Season—three sets of 8 to 12 reps, each side

2. Dumbbell Arm Swings

Purpose: To strengthen pectorals, shoulders, glutes, arms, abdominals, and core.

Basic: Dumbbell Arm Swings

Start by standing in a staggered-step position with feet about 12 inches apart, holding a dumbbell in each hand. With good posture, chest out and belly in, raise weights by bending at your elbows and keeping forearms mostly parallel to the ground, as shown in photo 28a. Simultaneously, pull one elbow straight back so your hand is underneath your armpit and other arm/elbow is forward, as in a running motion. Swing shoulders back and forth, maintaining good upright posture and pulling shoulders back. Reverse foot position halfway through the repetitions. (See page 60.)

Intermediate: Arm Swings with Stretch Cord

Same position as the Basic, except you will hold the ends of the stretch cord in each hand. Secure the stretch cord in a doorjamb so that you have two equidistant ends to the cord. Maintain a staggered position for half the number of repetitions, then switch staggered position with opposite leg and perform the remaining number of repetitions.

Advanced: Arm Swings with Stretch Cord Standing with Leg Raised

Same as the Intermediate, except you will stand on one leg with the other knee raised in front. Perform half the number of repetitions on one leg and then repeat the remaining number of repetitions on the opposite leg.

Sets/Reps: Off-Season—three sets of 8 to 12 reps

3. Jump Squats onto Step or Box

Purpose: To strengthen glutes, hamstrings, quads, ankles, abs, core, and balance.

Basic: Jump Squats onto Step or Box

Start in a standing position with your feet about shoulder-width apart in front of a step or box. With your arms at your sides, inhale and perform a deep squat. From the deep squat position exhale and jump onto the step or box with both feet, landing in a squat position. Step off step or box and repeat the squat and jump. (See page 50.)

Intermediate: Jump Squats onto BOSU

Same as the Basic, except you will start by standing in front of a BOSU and jump onto it, landing in a squat position. Step off the BOSU and perform the squat and jump again.

Advanced: Jump Squats on the BOSU

Start by standing on the BOSU. Perform a deep squat and jump by extending your legs, hips, and glutes straight up, landing in a deep squat position back on the BOSU. Repeat the jump and squat.

Sets/Reps: Off-Season—three sets of 8 to 12 reps

4. Side Lunge with Front Raise

Purpose: To strengthen glutes, hamstrings, quads, ab/adductors, shoulders, and core.

Basic: Side Lunge with Front Raise

Start in a standing position with a dumbbell in each hand at your sides. Perform a side lunge, keeping your hips back and lunging leg bent while your other leg stays straight. From that position raise your arms with dumbbells out straight to shoulder height, hold, and then simultaneously bring your arms back to your sides while extending your hips, glutes, and quads back to the start position. Perform half of the repetitions on one leg and then switch and perform half of the repetitions on the other leg. (See page 35.)

Intermediate: Side Lunge onto Step with Front Raise

Same as the Basic, except side-lunge onto a step.

Advanced: Side Lunge onto BOSU with One-Arm Front Raise

Same as the Intermediate, except side-lunge onto a BOSU so your foot strikes the center of it and raise the same side arm. Then, repeat with other leg and arm.

Sets/Reps: Off-Season—three sets of 8 to 12 reps

5. Obliques over BOSU

Purpose: To strengthen obliques and core.

Basic: Obliques over BOSU

Start by lying on the BOSU with the small of your back centered on top, both arms behind your head, and your feet on the floor. Slightly raise your torso off the BOSU while pointing one elbow toward the opposite knee. Hold and return to the start position, and then repeat with the opposite elbow toward the other knee. Repeat by alternating sides. (See page 51.)

Intermediate: Obliques over BOSU with One Leg Raised

Same as the Basic, except with both hands behind your head, slightly raise your torso while raising the left leg and pointing the right elbow toward the left knee. Outstretched leg should remain off the floor. Repeat on that side and then switch legs and repeat on the other side. (See page 52.)

Advanced: Bicycles over BOSU with Legs Raised

Same as the Intermediate, except with both hands behind your head, raise your torso and legs off the floor so you are balanced on the BOSU. Extend one leg straight and keep the other leg bent. Start the movement by bringing the knee of the extended leg to the opposite elbow so they make contact. Repeat this movement with the opposite arm and leg, alternating the movement from one side to the other while maintaining balance on the BOSU. (See page 52.)

Sets/Reps: Off-Season—three sets of 8 to 12 reps, each side

Second Phase: Preseason of Duathlete Program (reps increase to 10–12)

Once we are about eight to twelve weeks away from our first major race of the year, we will transition into the Preseason Phase of the Duathlete Program. This phase starts with the Fink Five and then goes right into the following three exercises, which most practiced athletes can complete in about 7.5 minutes. If an athlete starts with the Easy Eight warm-up routine (5 minutes), then completes the Fink Five (12 minutes), and then finishes up with the following three Preseason Exercises (7.5 minutes), he or she can complete the entire Preseason Program in less than 25 minutes.

1. Lateral Lunge/Squat across BOSU

Purpose: To strengthen glutes, hamstrings, quads, ankles, core, and balance, and to develop power.

Basic: Lateral Lunge/Squat across BOSU

Start by standing on the BOSU. Then, take one leg and lunge to the side into a deep squat, keeping your other foot on the BOSU. Then quickly jump your off foot onto the BOSU and lunge with the other leg to the opposite side. Repeat side to side quickly while maintaining good form. (See page 39.)

Intermediate: Lateral Lunge/Squat across BOSU with Medicine Ball Reach

Start by standing on the BOSU with a medicine ball at chest height, with bent arms. Take one leg and lunge to the side into a deep squat, keeping your other foot on BOSU, and simultaneously extend the medicine ball straight out in front. Bring the medicine ball back to your chest, and then quickly jump your off foot onto the BOSU and lunge with the other leg to the opposite side while reaching out front with the medicine ball again. Repeat side to side quickly while maintaining good form.

Advanced: Lateral Lunge/Squat across BOSU with 180° Turn

Start by standing on the BOSU. Take one leg and lunge to the side into a deep squat, keeping the other foot on the BOSU. Then quickly jump straight up with both legs and simultaneously make a 180° turn so you face the opposite direction, landing with the opposite foot on the BOSU and the other foot on the ground. Jump across the BOSU and repeat 180° turn on that side. Repeat side to side quickly with the 180° turn while maintaining good form. (See page 40.)

Sets/Reps: Preseason—three sets of 10 to 12 reps

2. One-Leg Press to Hop (with or without dumbbells)

Purpose: To strengthen glutes, hamstrings, quads, ankles, core, and balance, and to develop power.

Basic: One-Leg Press with Foot on Step (with or without dumbbells)

Start by standing in a lunge position with one foot on the step and the other foot behind, with knee bent almost to the floor. Perform a one-leg press with the leg on the step and rise to a standing position while bringing the opposite leg up with raised knee. Return to the start position and repeat on that leg and then switch to the other leg. (See page 40.)

Intermediate: One-Leg Press to Hop with Foot on Step (with or without dumbbells)

Same as the Basic, except after you complete the press, hop on the same leg while keeping the opposite leg raised in a chair pose. Return to the start position and repeat on the same leg before switching to the opposite leg for the remaining repetitions. (See page 41.)

Advanced: One-Leg Press to Hop with Foot on BOSU (with or without dumbbells)

Same as the Intermediate, except start with one foot on the BOSU. Then, after you complete the press, hop on that same leg while raising the opposite knee in a chair pose. Repeat on the same leg before switching to the opposite leg.

Sets/Reps: Preseason—three sets of 10 to 12 reps, each leg

3. Get-ups off BOSU with Arms at Your Sides

Purpose: To strengthen core and abdominals, glutes, quads, and hamstrings.

Basic: Get-ups off the BOSU with Arms at Your Sides

Start by sitting on the BOSU with arms at your sides and bent knees. Extend your torso back so you are completely parallel to the floor and legs are raised off the floor. Then, raise torso and simultaneously put your feet on the floor and stand straight up. Then, return to the start position and repeat. (See page 41.)

Intermediate: Get-ups off BOSU with Arms Raised

Same as the Basic, except with both arms extended over your head for the entire exercise. Raise your torso and simultaneously bring your feet to the floor and stand up, keeping arms extended over your head.

Advanced: Get-ups off Floor with Medicine Ball Overhead

Same as the Intermediate, except start by lying on the floor instead of the BOSU, with knees bent and holding a medicine ball over your head. As you begin to "get up," bring the ball down from over your head to in front of your chest.

Sets/Reps: Preseason—three sets of 10 to 12 reps

Third Phase: Competitive Season of Duathlete Program (reps increase to 12–15 range)

Once we have completed our first major race of the year, we will transition into the Competitive-Season Phase of the Duathlete Program. This phase starts with the Fink Five and then goes right into the following three exercises, which most practiced athletes can complete in about 7.5 minutes. If an athlete starts with the Easy Eight warm-up routine (5 minutes), then completes the Fink Five (12 minutes), and then finishes up with the following three Competitive-Season Exercises (7.5 minutes), he or she can complete the entire Competitive-Season Program in less than 25 minutes. Additional Note: As part of a proper pre-race taper, it is our general suggestion not to perform strength training during the week immediately preceding a major race.

1. Rear Deltoid Flys in Stork Position

Purpose: To strengthen deltoids, rhomboids, hamstrings, quads, core, and balance.

Basic: Rear Deltoid Flys in Stork Position

Start in a standing position with a dumbbell in each hand. Raise one leg straight behind you and balance on the other leg in a stork position, letting your arms hang straight down. Depress your shoulder blades toward your spine and raise the dumbbells with slightly bent arms out to the sides, but not higher than shoulder height. Hold for a 2-second count and then return arms back to the start position and repeat. Keep hands soft as you squeeze your shoulder blades together to elevate the weights. Perform half the repetitions on one leg and then switch and perform half the repetitions on the other leg. (See page 36.)

Intermediate: Rear Deltoid Flys in Stork Position, Alternating Arms

Same as the Basic, except perform this exercise by raising one arm at a time and alternating arms. Perform half of the repetitions on one leg and then switch and perform half of the repetitions on the other leg.

Advanced: Rear Deltoid Flys with One-Leg Squat in Stork Position

Same as the Basic, except start this exercise from the stork position and begin with a one-leg squat; then, as you extend from the squat, simultaneously raise the weights as you return to the start position. Perform half of the repetitions on one leg and then switch and perform half of the repetitions on the other leg.

Sets/Reps: Competitive Season—three sets of 12 to 15 reps

2. Superman on BOSU

Purpose: To strengthen back, shoulders, glutes, hamstrings, abdominals, and core.

Basic: Superman on BOSU

Start by lying facedown with your hips centered on the BOSU, your legs straight and hip-width apart, and your palms facing up. Extend your shoulder blades back and down toward your spine. Inhale to prepare for the movement and then exhale as you extend your lower back, squeezing your glutes as you extend your torso up while rotating your thumbs toward the ceiling. Hold for 1 second in that position before returning to the start position. (See page 44.)

Intermediate: Superman on BOSU with Arms Overhead

Same as the Basic, except raise your arms over your head and perform the movement without rotating your thumbs toward ceiling. (See page 44.)

Advanced: Swimming on BOSU

Start by lying facedown, balanced on your midsection over the BOSU, with legs extended and arms overhead. Raise your arms and legs off the floor, find your balance, and then perform a swimming-type movement (no need to do the crawl stroke, exactly) by fluttering your arms and legs for about 30 to 60 seconds. (See page 44.)

Sets/Reps: Competitive Season—three sets of 12 to 15 reps
Advanced: Sets/Reps: Competitive Season—three sets of 30 to 60 seconds

3. Overhead Raises with Stretch Cords or Bands

Purpose: To strengthen shoulders, back, lats, abdominals, and core.

Basic: Overhead Raises with Stretch Cords or Bands

Start by holding one end of a stretch cord in both hands and place your foot on the other end of the stretch cord on the floor to hold it in place. Give yourself enough slack so you can extend the stretch cord directly over your head, keeping your arms straight. While keeping your arms straight, raise the stretch cord directly above your shoulders and head; then, lower to start position and repeat.

Intermediate: Overhead Raises with Stretch Cords or Bands in Lunge Position

Same as the Basic, except stagger your feet in a lunge position while raising the stretch cord directly over your head. Split the repetitions between each leg. (See page 45.)

Advanced: Squat with Overhead Raises Using Kettle Bell

Start by standing with feet shoulder-width apart, holding one kettle bell with both hands. Begin by squatting back and bringing the kettle bell through your legs. Then, while extending out of the squat and returning to a standing position, simultaneously swing the kettle bell straight out in front and above your head while keeping your arms straight. Then, slowly lower the kettle bell and return to the start position. (See page 46.)

Sets/Reps: Competitive Season—three sets of 12 to 15 reps

Adventure Racer Program

This program includes the following exercises:

Off-Season	Preseason	Competitive Season
Fink Five	Fink Five	Fink Five
1. Ax Chop on BOSU	1. Side Lunge to	1. Get-ups off BOSU
2. Chest Flys	Front Raise	2. Overhead Raises
3. Squat, Curl, Press	2. One-Leg Press/Hop	3. Superman on BOSU
4. Rear Delt Flys	3. Side Planks	
5. Sliders to Side		

First Phase: Off-Season of Adventure Racer Program

In the Off-Season, the Adventure Racer Program starts with the Fink Five and then goes right into the following five exercises, which most practiced athletes can complete in 12 minutes. If an athlete starts with the Easy Eight warm-up routine (5 minutes), then completes the Fink Five (12 minutes), and then finishes up with the following five exercises (12 minutes), he or she can complete the entire program in less than 30 minutes.

1. Squat with Ax Chop on BOSU

Purpose: To strengthen hamstrings, quads, glutes, abdominals, arms, shoulders, and back.

Basic: Squat with Ax Chop on BOSU Using Medicine Ball

Start by standing on top of the BOSU and holding a medicine ball at shoulder height to one side, with arms bent. As you are performing a squat, and at the same pace as the squat, lower the medicine ball to the opposite side across your body in a chopping motion until you complete the squat. Return to the start position, extending the legs while reversing the chopping motion, and then repeat on the same side before switching to the other side. (See page 33.)

Intermediate: Squat with Ax Chop on BOSU Using Kettle Bell

Same as the Basic, except use a kettle bell to perform the exercise.

Advanced: Side Lunge with Ax Chop on BOSU Using Kettle Bell

Start by standing on top of the BOSU, holding a kettle bell at shoulder height to one side with arms bent. As you are performing a side lunge, swing the kettle bell to the opposite side across your body in a chopping motion to the outside of your lunging leg until you complete the lunge. Return to the start position and bring the kettle bell back to the opposite shoulder by reversing the chopping motion. Repeat on the opposite side.

Sets/Reps: Off-Season—three sets of 8 to 12 reps, each side

2. Chest Flys with Stretch Cords in Lunge Position

Purpose: To strengthen pectorals, shoulders, glutes, hamstrings, abdominals, core, and balance.

Basic: Chest Flys with Stretch Cords in Lunge Position

Start in a standing position holding the ends of the stretch cord in both hands, facing away from the door/wall with your legs in a lunge position. Extend your slightly bent arms out to the sides about chest level. Inhale, then exhale as you squeeze your chest and bring your arms together in front with palms facing down, hold, then return to the start position while keeping your arms extended from your sides. (See page 34.)

Intermediate: Chest Flys with Stretch Cords, Standing on One Leg

Same as the Basic, except start by standing on one leg. Perform the movement with one leg raised for half of the repetitions and then repeat with the other leg raised for the other half of the repetitions.

Advanced: Alternating Arm/Chest Flys with Stretch Cords, Standing on One Leg

Same as the Intermediate, except with leg raised, perform the movement with alternating arms. Start with both arms extended in front of you and then perform a fly with only one arm. Perform half of the repetitions on one leg and then switch legs and perform the remaining repetitions.

Sets/Reps: Off-Season—three sets of 8 to 12 reps

3. Squat to Curl and Press

Purpose: To strengthen glutes, hamstrings, biceps, shoulders, and core.

Basic: Squat to Curl and Press

Start in a standing position with a dumbbell in each hand. Begin by inhaling, and then perform a freestanding squat. As you return from the squat position, begin to curl the dumbbells as you get to the start position and then press the dumbbells over your head. Return the dumbbells to your sides and repeat. (See page 75.)

Intermediate: Squat on BOSU, Curl and Press

Same as the Basic, except start by standing on the BOSU.

Advanced: Squat on One Leg, Curl and Press

Same as the Basic, except start by raising one leg straight up with knee bent and parallel to the ground. Swing leg back, perform squat with other leg, then curl and press the weights over your head, and then return the weights to your sides. Repeat with same leg through a complete set of reps before switching to the other leg.

Sets/Reps: Preseason—three sets of 8 to 12 reps

4. Rear Deltoid Flys in Stork Position

Purpose: To strengthen deltoids, rhomboids, hamstrings, quads, core, and balance.

Basic: Rear Deltoid Flys in Stork Position

Start in a standing position with a dumbbell in each hand. Raise one leg straight behind you and balance on the other leg in a stork position, letting your arms hang straight down. Depress your shoulder blades toward your spine and raise the dumbbells with slightly bent arms out to the sides, but not higher than shoulder height. Hold for a 2-second count and then return arms back to the start position and repeat. Keep hands soft as you squeeze your shoulder blades together to elevate the weights. Perform half the repetitions on one leg and then switch and perform half the repetitions on the other leg. (See page 36.)

Intermediate: Rear Deltoid Flys in Stork Position, Alternating Arms

Same as the Basic, except perform this exercise by raising one arm at a time and alternating arms. Perform half of the repetitions on one leg and then switch and perform half of the repetitions on the other leg.

Advanced: Rear Deltoid Flys with One-Leg Squat in Stork Position

Same as the Basic, except start this exercise from the stork position and begin with a one-leg squat; then, as you extend from the squat, simultaneously raise the weights as you return to the start position. Perform half of the repetitions on one leg and then switch and perform half of the repetitions on the other leg.

Sets/Reps: Off-Season—three sets of 8 to 12 reps

5. Sliders to Side

Purpose: To strengthen ab/adductors, glutes, hamstrings, quads, abs, core, and balance.

Basic: Sliders to Side

This exercise is best performed on a hardwood floor or other semi-slick surface. Start in a standing position with a piece of paper under one foot. Begin by sliding the foot with the paper under it to the side, keeping the leg straight as you bend the opposite hip and knee into a lunge position. Use your glutes and hamstrings to return your leg next to other leg in a standing position. Repeat with that leg through a full set of repetitions, and then repeat with paper under the other foot. (See page 105.)

Intermediate: Sliders to Side (with dumbbells)

Same as the Basic, except hold a dumbbell in each hand while performing the movement.

Advanced: Sliders to Half-Circle (with dumbbells)

Start in staggered-stance position with a piece of paper under the foot in front (starting at twelve o'clock). Begin by sliding the front foot around in a half-circle all the way to the six o'clock position while bending at the hip and knee on the other leg. Repeat on that leg through a full set of repetitions and then repeat with paper under the other foot. To add difficulty, hold a dumbbell in each hand. (See page 105.)

Sets/Reps: Off-Season—three sets of 8 to 12 reps, each leg

Second Phase: Adventure Racer Program (reps increase to 10–12 range)

Once we are about eight to twelve weeks away from our first major race of the year, we will transition into the Preseason Phase of the Adventure Racer Program. This phase starts with the Fink Five and then goes right into the following three exercises, which most practiced athletes can complete in about 7.5 minutes. Therefore, if an athlete starts with the Easy Eight warm-up routine (5 minutes), then completes the Fink Five (12 minutes), and then finishes up with the following three Preseason Exercises (7.5 minutes), he or she can complete the entire Preseason Program in less than 25 minutes.

1. Side Lunge with Front Raise

Purpose: To strengthen glutes, hamstrings, quads, ab/adductors, shoulders, and core.

Basic: Side Lunge with Front Raise

Start in a standing position with a dumbbell in each hand at your sides. Perform a side lunge, keeping your hips back and lunging leg bent while your other leg stays straight. From that position raise your arms with dumbbells out straight to shoulder height, hold, and then simultaneously bring your arms back to your sides while extending your hips, glutes, and quads back to the start position. Perform half of the repetitions on one leg and then switch and perform half of the repetitions on the other leg. (See page 35.)

Intermediate: Side Lunge onto Step with Front Raise

Same as the Basic, except side-lunge onto a step.

Advanced: Side Lunge onto BOSU with One-Arm Front Raise

Same as the Intermediate, except side-lunge onto a BOSU so your foot strikes the center of it, and raise the same side arm. Then, repeat with other leg and arm.

Sets/Reps: Preseason—three sets of 10 to 12 reps / Advanced—three sets of 10 to 12 reps, each side

2. One-Leg Press to Hop (with or without dumbbells)

Purpose: To strengthen glutes, hamstrings, quads, ankles, core, balance, and power.

Basic: One-Leg Press with Foot on Step (with or without dumbbells)

Start by standing in a lunge position with one foot on the step and the other foot behind, with knee bent almost to the floor. Perform a one-leg press with the leg on the step and rise to a standing position while bringing the opposite leg up with raised knee. Return to the start position and repeat on that leg and then switch to the other leg. (See page 40.)

Intermediate: One-Leg Press to Hop with Foot on Step (with or without dumbbells)

Same as the Basic, except after you complete the press, hop on the same leg while keeping the opposite leg raised in a chair pose. Return to the start position and repeat on the same leg before switching to the opposite leg for the remaining repetitions. (See page 41.)

Advanced: One-Leg Press to Hop with Foot on BOSU (with or without dumbbells)

Same as the Intermediate, except start with one foot on the BOSU. Then, after you complete the press, hop on that same leg while raising the opposite knee in a chair pose. Repeat on the same leg before switching to the opposite leg.

Sets/Reps: Preseason—three sets of 10 to 12 reps, each leg

3. Side Planks

Purpose: To strengthen obliques, abdominals, core, and shoulders.

Basic: Side Plank on Floor

Start by lying on your side on the floor with your upper body resting on your bent elbow under your shoulder and your other arm at your side. Draw in your belly and hold while raising your hip and torso off the floor, with weight on your forearm, until there is a straight line from your ankles to your head. Hold for 5- to 10-second count and maintain drawn-in belly as you lower hips to the floor. Repeat on your other side. (See page 76.)

Intermediate: Side Plank on Floor with Arm Raise

Same as the Basic, except raise and lower your top arm repeatedly with palm facing up while holding the position for a 15- to 30-second count and then repeat on your other side.

Advanced: Side Plank on Floor with Ab Crunch

Same as the Basic, except place the hand of your top arm behind your head with bent elbow. While holding plank position, rotate your elbow toward the floor and repeat for the desired number of repetitions, and then repeat on your other side. (See page 77.)

Sets/Reps: Preseason—three sets of 10 to 12 reps, each side

Third Phase: Competitive Season of Adventure Racer Program (reps increase to 12–15 range)

Once we have completed our first major race of the year, we will transition into the Competitive-Season Phase of the Adventure Racer Program. This phase starts with the Fink Five and then goes right into the following three exercises, which most practiced athletes can complete in about 7.5 minutes. If an athlete starts with the Easy Eight warm-up routine (5 minutes), then completes the Fink Five (12 minutes), and then finishes up with the following three Competitive-Season Exercises (7.5 minutes), he or she can complete the entire Competitive-Season Program in less than 25 minutes. Additional Note: As part of a proper pre-race taper, it is our general suggestion not to perform strength training during the week immediately preceding a major race.

1. Get-ups off BOSU with Arms at Your Sides

Purpose: To strengthen core and abdominals, glutes, quads, and hamstrings.

Basic: Get-ups off the BOSU with Arms at Your Sides

Start by sitting on the BOSU with arms at your sides and bent knees. Extend your torso back so you are completely parallel to the floor and legs are raised off the floor. Then, raise torso and simultaneously put your feet on the floor and stand straight up. Then, return to the start position and repeat. (See page 41.)

Intermediate: Get-ups off BOSU with Arms Raised

Same as the Basic, except with both arms extended over your head for the entire exercise. Raise your torso and simultaneously bring your feet to the floor and stand up, keeping arms extended over your head.

Advanced: Get-ups off Floor with Medicine Ball Overhead

Same as the Intermediate, except start by lying on the floor instead of the BOSU, with knees bent and holding a medicine ball over your head. As you begin to "get up," bring the ball down from over your head to in front of your chest.

Sets/Reps: Competitive Season—three sets of 12 to 15 reps

2. Overhead Raises with Stretch Cords or Bands

Purpose: To strengthen shoulders, back, lats, abdominals, and core.

Basic: Overhead Raises with Stretch Cords or Bands

Start by holding one end of a stretch cord in both hands and place your foot on the other end of the stretch cord on the floor to hold it in place. Give yourself enough slack so you can extend the stretch cord directly over your head, keeping your arms straight. While keeping your arms straight, raise the stretch cord directly above your shoulders and head; then, lower to start position and repeat.

Intermediate: Overhead Raises with Stretch Cords or Bands in Lunge Position

Same as the Basic, except stagger your feet in a lunge position while raising the stretch cord directly over your head. Split the repetitions between each leg. (See page 45.)

Advanced: Squat with Overhead Raises Using Kettle Bell

Start by standing with feet shoulder-width apart, holding one kettle bell with both hands. Begin by squatting back and bringing the kettle bell through your legs. Then, while extending out of the squat and returning to a standing position, simultaneously swing the kettle bell straight out in front and above your head while keeping your arms straight. Then, slowly lower the kettle bell and return to the start position. (See page 46.)

Sets/Reps: Competitive Season—three sets of 12 to 15 reps

3. Superman on BOSU

Purpose: To strengthen back, shoulders, glutes, hamstrings, abdominals, and core.

Basic: Superman on BOSU

Start by lying facedown with your hips centered on the BOSU, your legs straight and hip-width apart, and your palms facing up. Extend your shoulder blades back and down toward your spine. Inhale to prepare for the movement and then exhale as you extend your lower back, squeezing your glutes as you extend your torso up while rotating your thumbs toward the ceiling. Hold for 1 second in that position before returning to the start position. (See page 44.)

Intermediate: Superman on BOSU with Arms Overhead

Same as the Basic, except raise your arms over your head and perform the movement without rotating your thumbs toward ceiling. (See page 44.)

Advanced: Swimming on BOSU

Start by lying facedown, balanced on your midsection over the BOSU, with legs extended and arms overhead. Raise your arms and legs off the floor, find your balance, and then perform a swimming-type movement (no need to do the crawl stroke, exactly) by fluttering your arms and legs for about 30 to 60 seconds. (See page 44.)

Sets/Reps: Competitive Season—three sets of 12 to 15 reps
Advanced: Sets/Reps: Competitive Season—three sets of 30 to 60 seconds

Special Travel Program

Here is a very simple program you can use while traveling. It requires only a stretch cord and can be adapted to your own level of fitness. It's designed for situations when an athlete finds him- or herself without the proper equipment and training facilities to complete any of the sport-specific programs in this book. The Special Travel Program can be done anywhere—even in a hotel room—and all you need to do is to remember to bring your stretch cord. Once practiced a few times, the Special Travel Program takes most athletes less than 20 minutes to complete.

The program consists of the following eight exercises:

1. Squats
2. Push-ups
3. One-Leg Squat with Row
4. Alternating-Arm Bicep Curls

5. One-Arm Tricep Extensions
6. Straight-Arm Overhead Raises
7. Planks
8. Side Planks with Hip Raises

1. Squats

Start by standing straight with feet about shoulder-width apart and hands behind your head. Begin the squat by bending at your hips and knees as you push back into a squat position, bringing your quadriceps as close to parallel to the floor as possible. Hold and then press through your heels as you extend your hips,

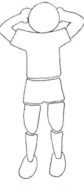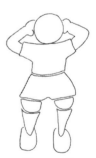

Figure 1   *Figure 2*

knees, and ankles, and return to the start position. Repeat for the desired number of repetitions. (See figures 1 and 2 above.)

Sets/Reps: Off-Season—three sets of 8 to 10 reps / Preseason—three sets of 10 to 12 reps / Competitive Season—three sets of 12 to 15 reps

2. Basic Bent-Knee or Straight-Leg Push-ups

Start with your knees or feet on the floor and arms straight and wider than shoulder-width apart. Keep spine neutral as you lower your chest toward the floor by bending your elbows. Hold and then return to the start position. For advanced push-ups, cross one leg over the other and perform the push-up on one leg only. (See figures 3 and 4, right.)

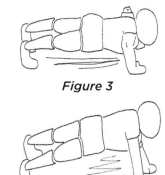

Figure 3

Sets/Reps: Off-Season—three sets of 8 to 12 reps / Preseason—three sets of 10 to 12 reps / In-Season—three sets of 12 to 15 reps

Figure 4

3. One-Leg Squat with Row Using Stretch Cord

Secure one end of the stretch cord in a doorjamb and close the door. Start by standing on your left leg with the stretch cord in your right hand. Stand far enough away from the door so that there is sufficient tension on the stretch cord. Then, with your left leg, flex at your knee and hip as you lower into a squat

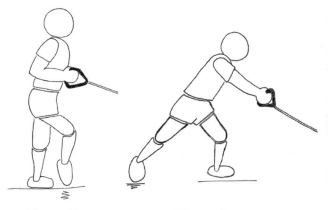

Figure 5　　　　　　*Figure 6*

position, keeping your right arm extended and straight. As you return to the start position, simultaneously pull the stretch cord straight back, bringing your elbow back so your hand is at about your lower ribs and your elbow is behind you. Hold that position, then repeat the one-leg squat and row again on that same side. Then, repeat on the right leg, holding the stretch cord in your left hand. (See figures 5 and 6 above.)

Sets/Reps: Off-Season—three sets of 8 to 10 reps, each leg/arm / Preseason—three sets of 10 to 12 reps, each leg/arm / Competitive Season—three sets of 12 to 15 reps, each leg/arm

4. Alternating-Arm Bicep Curls with Stretch Cords

Start with one end of the stretch cord in each hand and under both feet, about shoulder-width apart. With knees slightly bent, at a controlled speed, perform a full curl with one arm and then the other arm, and keep alternating arms. If you are in Preseason or Competitive Season, you can modify this exercise by doing the alternating curls in quick succession. (See figures 7 and 8, right.)

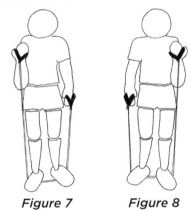

Figure 7   Figure 8

Sets/Reps: Off-Season—three sets of 8 to 12 reps, each arm / Preseason—three sets of 10 to 12 reps, each arm / Competitive Season—three sets of 12 to 15 reps, each arm

5. One-Arm Tricep Extension with Stretch Cords

Place one end of the stretch cord on the inside of a door and bring the other end along the floor and through the doorjamb, and close the door. Start by facing away from the door with one end of the stretch cord in one hand, with your arm bent behind you. From that starting position, stand tall as you extend your arm straight, hold, and then return to the

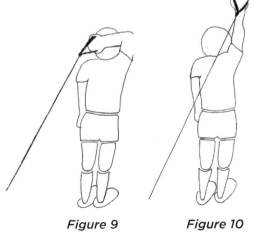

Figure 9   Figure 10

start position. Repeat for the desired number of repetitions with that arm,

134

then switch arms and repeat for the same number of repetitions on the other arm. (See figures 9 and 10 above.)

Sets/Reps: Off-Season—three sets of 8 to 10 reps, each arm / Preseason—three sets of 10 to 12 reps, each arm / Competitive Season—three sets of 12 to 15 reps, each arm

6. Straight-Arm Raises with Stretch Cords

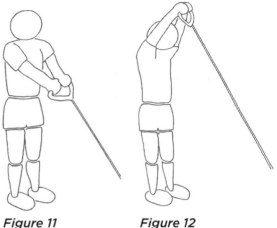

Place one end of the stretch cord on the inside of a door and bring the other end along the floor and through the doorjamb, and close the door. Hold one end of the stretch cord in both hands at about waist height. Then, with both hands and arms straight, extend the stretch cord straight up and over your head, directly above your shoulders. Hold and then return to the start position and repeat. (See figures 11 and 12 above.)

Figure 11　　　　　*Figure 12*

Sets/Reps: Off-Season—three sets of 8 to 12 reps / Preseason—three sets of 10 to 12 reps / Competitive Season—three sets of 12 to 15 reps

7. Planks

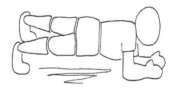

Start in a push-up position facedown on the floor, with your elbows under your shoulders and your forearms on the floor. Raise your body onto your toes and forearms, bringing your body in a straight line from your ankles to your shoulders. Keeping your back flat and holding your abdominals tight, hold that position for the desired number of seconds. (See figure 13 above.)

Figure 13

Sets/Reps: Off-Season—three sets of 30 to 60 seconds / Preseason—three sets of 45 to 60 seconds / Competitive Season—three sets of 60 to 90 seconds

8. Side Planks with Hip Raises

Start by lying on your side with your legs stacked on top of each other, your elbow bent under your shoulder, and your other arm straight at your side. Raise your hip off the floor and bring your body into a straight line from your ankles to your head. Hold that position for 2 to 3 seconds, and then repeat the hip raise for the desired number of repetitions on that side. Then, repeat the same thing on your other side. (See figures 14 and 15, right.)

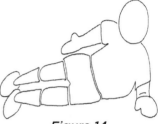

Figure 14

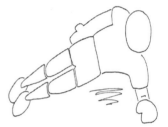

Figure 15

Sets/Reps: Off-Season—three sets of 8 to 12 reps, each side / Preseason—three sets of 10 to 12 reps, each side / Competitive Season—three sets of 12 to 15 reps, each side

CHAPTER 4

Drop the Excuses: Just Get Lean

Energy and persistence conquer all things.
—Benjamin Franklin

et's start with the simple truth about body weight: Your fastest body weight is likely to be your leanest healthy body weight. We have worked with hundreds of athletes over the years, and this maxim has been proven time and again. Surprisingly, many athletes either fail to grasp this simple truth or fail to act on it. The reality is that your body weight may be why your progress has stagnated.

In a way, it's a simple matter of power to weight. Any weight that does not help to propel your body forward or provide a necessary bodily function in support is just extra weight to carry. Ten pounds of excess fat around your middle is essentially the same as just carrying a ten-pound weight strapped to your middle. The weight doesn't help to propel your body forward, nor does it perform any needed bodily function. It's just extra weight being carried.

The Big Five Excuses

As coaches we hear a wide range of excuses on this topic. Some of the most common excuses and our typical responses to them are as follows:

1. I can't really eat well because I have children.
The "kids claim" is a weak excuse on two levels. First, it assumes that kids have to eat poorly. Second, it assumes that as their parent, you are forced to eat poorly, too. It all seems totally backwards to us. If they are your kids, shouldn't you make sure that they don't eat poorly? Shouldn't you be teaching them at an early age to eat healthfully? In fact, isn't one of the reasons you are an endurance athlete in the first place to help promote good health?

Setting the example of good nutrition for your family will greatly benefit your kids throughout their lives. They may not like it now, but they will thank you when they are healthy adults.

In Chapter 5, we will present several seven-day healthy eating plans that will not only help you to become healthier and leaner, but may also help your family to eat healthier, too.

2. I watch what I eat, but just can't seem to lose weight.
We usually hear this complaint from athletes who feel that they make wise food choices. They avoid fast food and junk food and try to eat healthy fruits, vegetables, and whole grains. Usually the issue here is not what these athletes are eating, but how much they are eating. In other words, they are making wise food choices, but they are not exercising good portion control.

Later in this chapter we will introduce some calorie-counting tools to help you add proper portion control to your already good diet.

3. If I lose too much weight I will feel weak.
Well, this much is true: Losing too much weight is not healthy. But, we usually hear this excuse from athletes who are not in any near-term risk of losing too much weight. Their body fat is higher than what it optimally should be. What they are really experiencing is low energy due to the cutting of calories.

Usually, this kind of low-energy athlete is only focusing on cutting calories and not on properly balancing the calories among carbohydrates, proteins, and fats, as well as properly timing their meals throughout the day. By not balancing and spacing meals properly, this kind of athlete experiences peaks and valleys in his or her energy level.

Later in this chapter we will present guidance to help you balance your calories properly, so you can enjoy a more-consistent energy level.

4. If I just train hard, my weight will take care of itself.
We hear this statement from athletes all the time. A variation on the theme occurs when people say something to us like, "I bet you can eat whatever you want since you train so much." We sure wish this were true, but unfortunately, it's not.

Most important, eating whatever you want won't give your body what it needs no matter how much you are training. Even if you trained for an average of 60 minutes per day—depending on your metabolic rate, the type of training, and your intensity level—you are likely to burn only between 600 and 1,000 calories. One trip to the fast-food drive-through will more than wipe out the calorie-burning benefits from that workout and prevent you from losing any weight.

There are really three key data points in determining what and how much you should eat to achieve your weight-loss goals: Calories consumed, calories utilized through exercise, and the calories required to maintain your body's normal function (i.e., basal metabolic rate, or BMR).

Later in this chapter we will discuss not only how to track these three variables, but also how to empower you to manage them throughout the day so that you can achieve your optimal body weight.

5. I eat out a lot and cannot seem to control what I eat.
It's very difficult to determine either the caloric content or the nutritional content of the food you eat when you eat out. Some athletes become pretty good at it, but the vast majority does not. Some smart athletes have certain "safe foods" they always try to order, and they ask questions of the server regarding the preparation of the food. But most of us are not very good at these things. In fact, most of us would be shocked to know the caloric content of some of the meals we have at restaurants.

So, where you get your meals generally comes down to a lifestyle choice. Serious athletes either need to limit how often they eat out so that they can better control caloric and nutritional intake, or they need to become well-educated and disciplined about exactly what and how much they eat when they do eat out.

If you hear yourself in any of the top five excuses above, don't worry. Obviously, you are not alone. But realize that to perform at your best and fully achieve your potential as an endurance athlete, you must fuel and hydrate with proper nutrition and achieve optimal body weight. This is the simple truth, and if you are serious, you need to drop the excuses and put a plan in place. The following information presented in this chapter will help you do just that.

There is a wealth of wonderful nutritional resources out there to help endurance athletes eat healthfully and achieve optimal racing weight. The frequent problem, however, is that these resources are just too complicated, too technical, or require too much time to plan. Athletes often tell us that they have read this or that book on nutrition and learned a lot of interesting information, but that it was either too complicated or too time-consuming to put into action. Then, they usually give out a big sigh and say, "Coach, can you just tell me what to eat?"

As in our previous books, we try to present information here in a straight-forward, easy-to-use format. We try to tell the athlete exactly what he or she needs to do to get the desired results, as opposed to writing about a lot of theory or getting into a lot of technical lingo. What follows in this chapter is a simple-to-use approach to healthy eating that has worked well for many of our coached athletes over the years. In Chapter 5 we present several seven-day menus that the athlete can put to immediate good use.

Take a Look at the Great Ones

We need to look no further than the top athletes in our individual sports to see that a lean, healthy body weight is important. The American council on Exercise (ACE) indicates that an acceptable percentage of an individual's weight to be comprised of fat is 25 to 31 percent for women and 18 to 25 percent for men. However, when it comes to athletes, the council identifies the range as being 14 to 20 percent for women and 6 to 13 percent for men. What we have seen working with endurance athletes for many years is that the elite among them gravitate toward the lower half of the athlete ranges.

While we are not saying that all endurance athletes need to be at the levels of these elite athletes, we would suggest that an endurance athlete should consider it important to be in the range for athletes, and perhaps, through the techniques presented in this chapter, find their optimal body weight.

Before starting any diet or nutrition plan, we encourage you to seek the advice of a competent nutrition expert. Let us say right up front that while we are certified personal trainers, we are not certified nutritional experts. What we talk about in this chapter is based on our personal experience working with our own training and nutrition, as well as the feedback we have received from the athletes we have worked with over the past many years. So, please consider what we have to say, but before starting your own plan, seek guidance from a certified professional.

AN IRONFIT MOMENT

If you need proof that our leanest healthy body weig
fastest body weight, you need look no further than an athlete's
VO2Max, which is a popular test that determines an athlete's ability
to process oxygen and convert it to energy. While having a high
VO2Max is partially genetic, proper training can increase one's
VO2Max. The top elite endurance athletes typically have a very
high VO2Max.

The simplest way for an average athlete to improve his or her
VO2Max is to lose weight. That's right; if all the other variables
remain the same, simply losing body weight raises VO2Max. This
makes sense if you think about it. If a racing car's engine remains
the same size, but you reduce the weight of the car, the speed of
the car increases.

Six-Meals-a-Day Approach

We have worked with hundreds of athletes for many years, helping them to
achieve optimal racing body weight. We have also seen athletes try many of
the seemingly endless approaches to weight loss that continually come and
go.

What we have observed is that the best way for most athletes to approach
their nutrition is to adopt a simple six-meals-a-day approach. Instead of the
traditional three big meals a day, eat six mini meals spread throughout the
day. This does not necessarily mean increasing your calories (although it
may in certain situations), but it does mean spreading your calories out more
evenly through your day.

There are two key advantages to taking this approach. First, you are giving your body the calories it needs when it needs them. Second, it keeps
your energy level higher and more consistent throughout the day, avoiding
periods of feeling tired and sluggish while your body is digesting a big meal.

One of the most common mistakes we see is athletes neglecting to consume calories before and after early-morning training sessions. While this
is bad enough, some athletes don't even hydrate before a morning workout.

The usual excuses are that they don't want that full feeling before training or that they are tight on time and would rather try to catch up on their nutrition later in the day. Or there's the classic one we love: "If I don't eat before my morning workout, I will burn more fat."

It is not true that an athlete burns more fat by not eating prior to a morning workout. In fact, such an approach actually encourages more body fat storage. While we are sleeping, our bodies are fasting. If our last calorie intake was around 7 p.m. on the previous day and we wake up at 5 a.m., then we have already fasted for ten hours. We dress, warm up, and go for a run, adding another two hours to this period.

What many athletes don't understand is that certain metabolic changes occur in our bodies, changes that have profound consequences on the rest of the day. If we put our bodies into a regular pattern of fasting for fourteen hours a day and eating during ten hours of the day, our bodies may become more efficient at storing fat during the ten hours to sustain us through the fourteen hours of not eating. Teaching our bodies to be good at storing fat is definitely not what we want to do.

Some athletes take morning fasting even further by waiting to eat until they get to work, which may be two to three hours from the time they wake up. Worse yet is the athlete who then eats something like a bagel and coffee—not a very balanced meal. This athlete has extended the fasting period from fourteen hours to eighteen to twenty hours. So, after he or she eats that first meal of the day, this athlete is famished by the time lunch rolls around and then overeats as a result. This creates a cycle of energy highs and lows throughout the day and into the evening.

While such an example may seem extreme, it's much more common than you may think. We see athletes following this type of pattern, or something close to it, on a regular basis. In fact, this is pretty much the pattern Don followed throughout most of his twenties. He is far too familiar with it, and its negative effects.

Late or nonexistent morning meals followed by a few large meals later in the day leads to the following:

- Low energy level for much of the day, which has a negative impact on training performance, work performance, and general mood.
- Excess and unwanted body fat, most often around the middle for men and in the thigh area for women.

- Generally unhealthy nutrition and greater risk for illness and injury.

The good news is that there is an easy fix for this situation. It's the six-meals-a-day approach we mentioned above. It's doable for virtually everyone, although it requires a definite change in how you view nutrition. But if you are a serious endurance athlete—and we suspect you are if you're reading this book—then it's a change you can make.

When we have worked with athletes to change them over to the six-meals-a-day approach, they have experienced the following benefits:

- Consistently higher energy level throughout the day, with positively impacted training performance, work performance, and general mood.
- Reduced feeling of hunger and cravings.
- Less body fat and an overall leaner physique.
- Generally healthier nutrition and less illness and injury.

Following is an example of one day in the life of one of our coached athletes who follows the six-meals-a-day approach:

5:00 a.m.	Wake up and early-morning healthy snack
5:30 to 6:30 a.m.	Run training session
7:30 a.m.	Mini breakfast
10:00 a.m.	Mid-morning healthy snack
12:30 p.m.	Mini lunch
3:30 p.m.	Mid-afternoon healthy snack
4:30 to 5:30 p.m.	Functional strength and core workout
6:30 p.m.	Mini dinner
10:00 p.m.	Bedtime

In the example above, there exists a pretty consistent interval of 2.5 to 3 hours between meals, not counting possible additional calories consumed during the two training sessions (i.e., the morning run and the afternoon strength-training session).

While the athlete in this example does not train into the evening, many athletes do. If an athlete does train in the evening, then a healthy snack of carbohydrates and protein shortly after training to help speed recovery is suggested. We will cover in detail exactly what athletes should eat and drink before, during, and after training sessions in later chapters.

Balancing Carbohydrates, Proteins, and Fats with Each Meal

So far we have talked about spreading out our caloric intake by having six smaller meals spaced evenly throughout the day. Now let's talk about what these meals should consist of.

In the example of the poor eater, after fasting all night and most of the morning, the athlete has a bagel and coffee to hold him over until lunch. This is not a very balanced meal, but rather an attempt to benefit from the stimulating effects of the coffee and the short-term energy from the carbohydrate-rich bagel. He is mostly tricking his body temporarily as opposed to truly fueling it.

The problem with just eating simple carbohydrates like those found in a bagel is that they provide a relatively short-range burst of energy. You feel the energy for a little while, but soon your energy level falls back to being as low as it was before, if not even lower. This fatigue is also usually accompanied by feelings of hunger, and even cravings for certain types of food. Now we're looking at typical days of energy highs and lows in a yo-yo pattern.

Such patterns are definitely not optimal for you as an athlete, and will probably also be a negative for your work performance and mood.

The best approach to having an even and consistent energy level throughout the day is not only spreading your daily food intake into six meals, but, to the extent possible, balancing those meals more evenly among carbohydrates, proteins, and fats. Over the years there have been many unbalanced diet fads: high-carbohydrate diets, low-carbohydrate diets, fat-free diets, etc. Many of these diets have short-term results, but as soon as the diet is over, the individual gains most (if not all) of the weight back.

The approach that really works, the one that can be maintained for life, is a well-balanced diet with proper portion control. What we mean by *balanced* is that our consumption of calories should be properly allocated between carbohydrates, proteins, and fats. For most people, the proper ratios are about 40 percent carbohydrates, 30 percent protein, and 30 percent fat. Most people maintain a more-even and consistently good energy level if

AN IRONFIT MOMENT

Keep in mind that all carbohydrates, proteins, and fat are not the same. We want our diets to be rich in healthy carbohydrates, proteins, and fats to make up an overall healthy diet. What does the USDA consider to be a healthy diet? The Dietary Guideline for Americans describes a healthy diet as one that:

- emphasizes fruits, vegetables, whole grains (complex rather than simple carbohydrates);
- contains fat-free or low-fat milk and milk products;
- includes lean meats, poultry, fish, beans, eggs, and nuts;
- and is low in saturated fats, trans fats, cholesterol, salt (sodium), and added sugars.

The healthy eating plans in Chapter 5 keep these guidelines in mind and include healthy examples of carbohydrates, fats, and protein.

they consume their calories in these general ratios. Furthermore, a nutritionally balanced eater will not suffer from cravings, which lead to binge eating and poor food choices.

These ratios may vary from athlete to athlete. Doing our own testing over time, we have found that while Melanie does her best with these ratios, Don does better with a little more carbohydrates and a little less fat than the 40 percent carbohydrates, 30 percent protein, and 30 percent fats ratios. He seems to perform best on ratios closer to 50 percent carbohydrates, 25 percent protein, and 25 percent fats. So, we encourage our coached athletes to track this over time, starting with the ratios of 40 percent carbohydrates, 30 percent protein, and 30 percent fats, and then testing and adjusting to determine what ratios help them to feel their best, maintain a high energy level, and perform optimally.

It is also important to note that these ratios are exclusive of additional calories consumed by endurance athletes immediately before, during, and after training. We will discuss these additional intakes in greater detail in Chapter 7, which is specifically about fueling for performance. As we will discuss, these "fueling" calories are mostly in the form of carbohydrates.

Because of fueling, many endurance athletes actually have overall (daily diet plus calories consumed right before, during, and after training and racing) carbohydrate ratios closer to 60 percent of total calories. But for now, we are focusing solely on an athlete's daily calorie consumption outside of those consumed immediately before, during, or after training.

The key for us as endurance athletes is to marry the six-meals-a-day approach with the balanced carbohydrate, protein, and fats approach.

In Chapter 5, we present several seven-day healthy eating plans for you to use as guidelines to help with your own meal planning. Each of these plans includes a rough 40 percent, 30 percent, and 30 percent balance of carbohydrates, protein, and fat, respectively.

Counting Calories

So, all we need to do is eat six meals a day and make sure that all of these meals are fairly balanced in carbohydrates, proteins, and fats, right? Well, while this is a great start, there's something else we need to take into account: portion control, or the number of calories we consume. You didn't really think we were going to talk about achieving and maintaining our optimum healthy body weight without talking about calorie counts, did you?

The simple truth is that we all have a unique number of calories that power our body's functions. This number is known as our *basal metabolic rate* (BMR). Stated simply, it's the number of calories we need to consume each day to allow our bodies to function normally and to maintain our current body weight. The BMR does not take into account any additional physical activity; it's just what is needed to cover basic function. Picture a normal healthy person who chooses to watch television in bed all day and have his meals brought to him.

Even without including our calories burned in training, our true daily calories burned are typically substantially higher than our BMR. Even when athletes are not training, they don't watch television in bed all day and have their food brought to them. They are going to work, cleaning the house, going shopping, walking the dog, and performing an endless list of other daily activities.

What we have found through our testing and working with many athletes over the years is that these activities typically equate to about 30 percent over their calculated BMR. We therefore like to focus on what we call "Active BMR," which is an estimation of the athlete's complete calorie needs, except for those burned in training.

One of the most generally accepted formulas for determining BMR is the Harris-Benedict Equation (originally published by James Arthur Harris and Francis Gano Benedict in 1919):

- BMR for Women: 655 + (4.35 x weight in pounds) + (4.7 x height in inches) – (4.7 x age in years)
- BMR for Men: 66 + (6.23 x weight in pounds) + (12.7 x height in inches) – (6.8 x age in years)

Following is Melanie's current BMR based on this formula:

BMR= 665 + (4.35 x 118 pounds) + (4.7 x 66.5 inches) – (4.7 x 46 years) = 1,275 calories

To determine Melanie's Active BMR, we will increase this result by 30%:

Active BMR: = 1,275 calories x 130% = 1,658 calories

What have we estimated here? If Melanie just did her normal activities and did not do any training, she would maintain her current weight by averaging about 1,658 calories taken in per day. We have tested this specific Active BMR for Melanie, as we have for many other athletes, and we have found that for these types of active people, this formula approach holds true.

A very popular weight-management method that athletes have used to either increase or decrease their body weight is the 500-calorie-per-day assumption. It's based on the fact that one pound is the equivalent of 3,500 calories, which, divided by seven days in a week, equals 500 calories per day. If an athlete increases his net calorie intake by about 500 calories a day over his Active BMR, he will typically gain about a pound per week. Likewise, if he decreases his average net calorie intake by an average of about 500 calories a day, he will typically lose about a pound per week.

If we want to lose body weight in an effort to get down to our optimal healthy body weight, we can plan around a 500-calorie reduction per day and then gradually lose about a pound per week until we achieve our goal.

A pound per week is a good rate at which to lose weight for most average-size athletes (although we will suggest an alternative approach for larger and smaller athletes later in this chapter). Many of the popular fad diets have you losing weight much faster, and it may not be healthy weight loss. If we lose weight gradually while training and eating properly, we are likely to reduce our body fat and retain more of our lean muscle. In other words, we lose the bad and keep the good.

If we lose weight very rapidly, however, we are more likely to lose good weight and bad weight at the same time. This is not what we want. We want to lose weight in a way that makes us leaner, healthier, and more energized—not weaker, less healthy, and run-down. Many people make this mistake.

So, for example, if an athlete with Melanie's Active BMR of 1,658 wanted to lose weight at a rate of one pound per week, one possible way to do it would be to pursue a 1,158-calorie-per-day target.

Target Calories per Day: 1,658 Adjusted BMR – 500 calories = 1,158 calories

Say it's the first week in January and the athlete is currently ten pounds heavier than she was a year ago when she set a new personal best time for the marathon. She wants to get back to that weight for the Boston Marathon coming up on the third Monday in April, which is about fifteen weeks away. This athlete can easily target a 500-calorie-per-day reduction in her calorie intake and be down to race weight several weeks in advance of her race. A 500-daily-calorie reduction is likely to result in the loss of a pound per week, which would have her down about ten pounds in ten weeks.

The 11 Calories per Pound Shortcut

We know that unless you went to engineering school or the like, the formulas discussed above may not be your cup of tea. Here's a great shortcut that we have found works better for many athletes. It's based on the estimation that to maintain our weight and cover our daily activities (i.e., Active BMR), we need to consume about 14 calories per pound of body weight per day, and to lose weight at a healthy rate of decrease, we need to consume about 11 calories per pound of body weight per day.

Many nutritional experts suggest a reasonable daily target of 10 calories per pound of body weight for most people trying to lose weight. But that figure applies to heavier, if not obese, sedentary people. Through our work with endurance athletes who are just looking to sculpt their bodies down to race weight, we find that a daily target of 11 calories per pound of body weight is usually optimal.

As an example, let's apply this guideline to Melanie.

Maintain Current Weight (Active BMR): 118 pounds x 14 calories = 1,652 calories

Reduce Weight at a Healthy Rate: 118 pounds x 11 calories = 1,298 calories

Note how close these results are to those calculated using the BMR formulas above. The Active BMR is almost identical (i.e., 1,652 vs. 1,658), and the targeted calorie number (1,298 vs. 1,158) is still fairly close.

While we have seen that both mathematical guidelines can be helpful for athletes, we actually prefer the "11 calories per pound" approach over the "subtract 500 calories" approach. It applies a consistent ratio (i.e., 11 calories for every one pound of body weight) to athletes of all weights, as opposed to applying a fixed number of calories (i.e., 500) to athletes of all weights, no matter how heavy or how light. For heavy athletes, 500 calories may not be enough, and for lighter athletes, it may be too much. Accordingly, we have found the "11 calories per pound" approach is most helpful to a wider range of athletes.

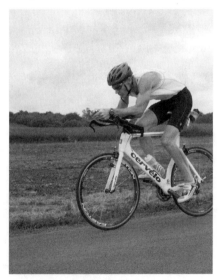

Net Calories from Training

So far, this weight management all seems doable enough. We need to adopt the six-meals-a-day approach, balance our meals properly with carbohydrates, proteins, and fats, and, if needed, we can gradually adjust our body weight by using either the "11 calories per pound" approach or the "subtract 500 calories from Active BMR" approach. Now, there is one

Elite 50-plus cyclist and endurance athlete Jeff Kellogg
Photo by Lynn Kellogg/ www.trilifephotos.com

more key element we need to add to the calculation to bring it all together: We need to net out the calories used in training.

In other words, while our Active BMR tells us the amount of calories we need to take in to maintain our current body weight, while performing our normal bodily functions and our regular daily activity, it does not take into account the large number of calories utilized by most endurance athletes in their daily training. If you like to eat, this is very good news.

So, for example, if your Active BMR is 1,650 and you typically utilize 800 calories every day by running for an hour a day, you will actually need to consume about 2,450 calories a day to maintain your current body weight.

Targeted Calories to Maintain Current Weight:

1,650 calories (Active BMR) + 800 calories utilized in training = 2,450 calories

Like we said, this is good news for those of us who enjoy eating a lot more than just 1,650 calories per day.

Now, what if the athlete wants to use this information to help "get down to race weight" at a safe rate of decrease, one that primarily loses fat and retains lean muscle?

The 118-pound athlete can use either the "subtract 500 calories" approach or the "11 calories per pound" approach as follows:

"Subtract 500 Calories" Approach:

1,650 calories (Active BMR) + 800 training calories – 500 calories = 1,950 calories

If this athlete continues to utilize about 800 calories per day in training, she needs to target daily calorie intake at about 1,950 in order to lose about one pound per week.

"11 Calories per Pound" Approach:

11 calories x 118 pounds + 800 calories = 2,098 calories

As per our comments above, we would typically suggest this approach for this particular athlete. Since she is lighter than average, the "subtract 500 calories" approach may be a bit too aggressive. We would suggest she target the 2,098 calories per day calculated by the "11 calories per pound" approach.

AN IRONFIT MOMENT

The most helpful technique we have used to help reduce our appetites is to drink one to two (depending on the body size of the athlete) 8-ounce glasses of water before all meals. Not *with* all meals, but *before* all meals. There is a big difference. There is a time delay between when we first consume food and/or hydration and when we actually experience the feeling of being full. By drinking one to two glasses of water before you start to eat, it gives your body time to feel fuller and decreases your appetite. This technique really works, and since endurance athletes need proper hydration anyway, the approach serves a dual purpose.

Estimating Calories for Athletic Activity

There are many good resources to help estimate the number of calories you utilize during the athletic activities in which you train. The American Council on Exercise's *Personal Trainer Manual* is one such source. Keep in mind that the number of calories one utilizes during training varies based on body mass, fitness level, genetics, and the intensity level of the exercise. Our suggestion is to determine general ranges for each activity in which you participate based on these factors, and then use them to properly estimate your calories utilized in training.

There are many helpful "calories burned" calculators available. Typically, you just need to input your weight, activity, duration, and intensity level, and a calculator will provide you with an estimation of your calories burned. Three of our favorite resources for these calculations are the following:

Health Status: healthstatus.com
Live Strong: livestrong.com
My Fitness Pal: myfitnesspal.com

In addition to the above resources, there are many other potential sources for this type of information. There are many heart rate monitors and other devices (like those produced by Garmin and Polar) that provide estimates of calories burned. Many exercise machines will do the same. Some of these sources provide very specific information, while others provide more general information. Double-check your sources to make sure you are getting reliable calorie information.

Following are typical hourly calorie-utilization ranges (from less vigorous effort to most vigorous effort) for an average-size athlete for some of the most common forms of physical activity:

Running: 600 to 1,000
Cycling: 500 to 900
Swimming: 400 to 800
Strength Training: 200 to 400

Melanie, who only weighs about 118 pounds, has determined her own unique hourly calorie-burning ranges to be the following:

Running: 600 to 800
Cycling: 500 to 700
Swimming: 400 to 600
Strength Training: 200 to 300

She therefore assigns a calorie amount within the range based on her heart rate or perceived level of intensity (less vigorous to most vigorous).

So, for example, if she has a very easy run she may assign it 600 calories per hour. But, if she were racing a half marathon, she may assign it 800 calories per hour.

Okay, we hear you; now it's getting a little more complicated. We have a six-meals-a-day eating plan; we are properly balancing our food consumption among carbohydrates, proteins, and fats; we are targeting specific daily calorie targets to gain, lose, or maintain our body weight; and we are netting out the number of calories per day utilized in training. That can be a lot to manage, so we suggest using one of the many great online applications.

Following are a few of our favorite calorie-counting (or equivalent) websites for your consideration:

loseit.com
myfitnesspal.com
weightwatchers.com

Calorie-Counting Example

The following is an example of an athlete's daily calorie calculation. This athlete has an Active BMR of 2,200 and wants to target a daily calorie reduction of 500 calories below this amount (i.e., 2,200 – 500 = 1,700) to achieve a weight loss of about one pound per week. She has estimated the calories for her six meals that day, as well as her estimated calories utilized in her training session that day. The athlete has successfully managed her calories throughout the day to achieve her net daily calorie target of 1,700:

Daily Calorie Example

Athlete: Kari Kona
Date: 1/28/14
Daily net calorie target: 1,700

Calories Consumed:

Meal #1:	350
Meal #2:	450
Meal #3:	350
Meal #4:	550
Meal #5:	350
Meal #6:	450
Total Calories Consumed (Total of Meals 1–6):	2,500
(Minus) Total Calories Utilized in Training:	-800
Net Daily Calories:	1,700

"Reward Foods"

For many years we have encouraged our coached athletes to designate certain foods as "reward foods." It's not practical to ban yourself totally from foods that you really enjoy. We may say we will, but eventually we are likely to give in. A much more practical approach is just to change our approach to them in a positive way. Instead of completely banning ourselves from a certain food, we will designate it as a reward food and only enjoy it when we have truly "earned" it.

Don's favorite junk food is french fries, and he usually enjoys them the most with plenty of salt. He knows this is not a good and healthy food, but he also knows that he would be fooling himself if he promised never to eat them again. A better approach is to designate french fries as a reward food, and only to enjoy them when he really feels like he has earned a reward. For Don, that usually means after a race, or sometimes after a very big and successful weekend of training. In fact, after a race, it's pretty much Don's ritual to hit a drive-through on the way home. By doing this, Don only eats french fries on occasion, and as part of a little celebration. Not only does this work

AN IRONFIT MOMENT

The Importance of Water and the "Pee Test"

Water is the most important nutrient. We all know that it's essential to maintain healthy levels of hydration each and every day, not only when we are training and racing. But experts do not always agree on exactly how much water we should consume outside of training.

The popular old rule of thumb is that the average-size male should consume about eight 8-ounce glasses of water per day, which is equal to 64 ounces (one gallon). In more recent years it has become the general consensus that this is probably on the low side for most, and that higher levels than this are preferred, especially for athletes and active people.

Our suggestion is to 1) follow the suggestions for proper hydration for before, during, and after training and racing as presented in Chapter 6; and 2) for the portions of the day when you are not training, start with the eight 8-ounce glasses per day approach, but then add or subtract from this amount based on the "pee test." Generally, the darker your urine is in color, the more dehydrated you are, and the clearer your urine is, the more hydrated you are. Ideally, you would like slightly yellow urine but not necessarily colorless. Use this simple test to help determine what daily hydration levels are best for you.

great from an overall healthy eating lifestyle, but it also works well mentally from a motivational standpoint. Looking forward to a reward like this after the race adds to the whole wonderful experience of racing.

Our suggestion is to try to live with a diet of balance and proportion. Designate certain foods as reward foods, and don't allow them to be part of your normal daily diet. In fact, don't even have them in your home. Why risk the temptation? Eat healthfully and save the reward food for when you truly deserve a reward.

In summary, there are four key elements to finding and maintaining your optimal healthy racing body weight:

- the six-meals-a-day approach;
- balancing meals between carbohydrates, fats, and protein;
- targeting and tracking your calories; and
- accounting for calories utilized in training and racing.

We hope you find our comments on healthy eating to be helpful. As we said in the beginning, please consider what we say here, but before taking action, consult a certified nutritional expert. Always be safe, proceed with caution, and put good health first.

CHAPTER 5

Your Optimal Healthy Eating Plan

> We are still masters of our fate. We are still
> captains of our souls.
>
> —*Winston Churchill*

For years we have heard from endurance athletes that they would like specific healthy eating plans. While we prefer to arm athletes with the tools and knowledge to develop their own diets, we understand why many athletes simply say, "Coach, it's too complicated, and I'm too busy to figure it all out; can you just tell me what to eat?"

If this is how you feel, then this chapter is for you. If you are just looking for ideas of foods to eat, or how often and how many calories to eat, these plans offer a lot of variety and sample foods. We present five seven-day healthy eating plans, each based on a targeted daily calorie level.

As we noted earlier in this book, we are not certified nutritionists. The plans we present here are based on what has worked well for many of the hundreds of athletes with whom we have worked over the years. Since everyone is different, we suggest playing it safe and reviewing any healthy eating plan— those offered here or elsewhere—with a nutritionist prior to starting it.

Selecting the Best Plan for You

To determine which of the five plans is best for you, you must first determine if you want to maintain your current weight, or if you want to lose weight. Once you make that decision, use either the "Active BMR" formula or the "calories per pound" methods presented in Chapter 4 to determine your targeted daily calories. Once you have made that determination, you can then select the plan that comes closest to your daily calorie level, with or without exercise.

For example, let's say you determined that your daily net calorie target should be 2,000, and that your average calories expended while exercising is about 500 per day. If that's the case, the 2,500 daily calories plan may be the best plan for you.

2,500 calories consumed – 500 calories expended in exercise = 2,000 net daily calories.

Another option may be to select the 2,250 daily calories plan because you typically supplement your daily nutrition with additional fueling and hydration calories that you consume before, during, or after exercise. For example, you may consume an energy gel (100 calories) and an energy drink (150 calories) before and/or during exercise.

2,250 calories from meals + 250 calories from energy gels and drinks – 500 calories expended during exercise = 2,000 net daily calories

These are just two possible ways to work with these plans to reach your daily calorie targets. We have some coached athletes who like to add a snack to a particular plan if they need extra calories to achieve their daily target.

Other coached athletes like to jump back and forth between plans since the length of their workouts varies, depending on the day. For example, they may work with the 1,500-calorie plan during the week when their workouts are shorter, and the 2,500-calorie plan on the weekend when their workouts are longer. There are many ways to use these plans to zero in on your exact daily-calories target.

We suggest you start simple by following just one of the plans, taking some time to get familiar with it and developing your own approach to modifying the plans based on what works best for you.

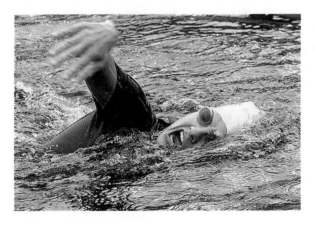

Melanie Fink competing in Ultraman Canada
Photo by Rick Kent

Special Dietary Requirements

Many of our athletes—such as our vegetarian, vegan, gluten-free, peanut-allergy, and diabetic clients—have special dietary requirements. We always recommend that these clients work with a certified nutritionist to understand how best to fulfill their dietary needs. However, we present some suggestions for substitutions within our plans that may be helpful.

For our vegetarian (non-vegan) athletes, it is very important to focus on getting sufficient daily protein intake. You can swap out the meats included in any of the five seven-day plans with alternative complete-protein substitutions, such as the following:

- Rice with beans
- Rice with sesame seeds
- Whole-wheat pasta with cheese
- Peanut butter with whole-wheat bread
- Lentil soup with cheese and whole-wheat bread
- Cereal with milk
- Tofu (legume) with cashews
- Quinoa (complete protein) with vegetables

These combinations are good substitutions because they provide a complete protein. Another option for some athletes is dairy products, which are also a complete protein.

Be sure to measure your servings to ensure that you have the proper portion and calories desired for any particular meal. For example, you may know that nuts are very high in calories, and it's always best to get out the measuring cup to accurately determine your calories.

These vegetarian substitutes, other than the whole-wheat pasta, apply to our gluten-free athletes, as well. For cereals, you will want to make sure they are rice- or corn-based, and again, be sure you observe the calories per serving size. Typically, what we have found is that gluten-free cereals are high in calories and the serving size is less than one cup.

Additionally, for our gluten-free athletes, there are many energy bars and fueling supplements that you can use before, during, and after training, such as the following:

- GU Chomps, Gels, and Energy Drink (guenergy.com)
- Bonk Breaker Energy Bars (bonkbreaker.com)
- KIND Bars (kindsnacks.com)
- Larabars (larabar.com)
- SOYJOY (soyjoy.com)
- LUNA Protein (clifbar.com)

Tips for Getting Started

We all know that maintaining good health through nutrition is vital for our success in endurance sports. And no, it's not an easy task. It takes time, planning, and discipline to fuel your body, but it can and should be done.

So, where to start? The following tips may help you on the road toward achieving your ultimate nutrition plan.

- Find a space in the pantry or cabinet that you can designate as your own. If your partner is willing to join as well, empty your pantry of items you no longer want in your new plan.
- Select a nutrition plan that you think will work for you. Review it and find the foods that you absolutely will not eat and substitute them with something else. Copy the plan and post it on your refrigerator, with the first day on top.
- From that plan make a shopping list and head to the supermarket and get your basic staples to achieve your seven-day nutrition plan. Remember the limes and lemons for your water.
- Set up your pantry and refrigerator with your new foods and arrange them by day.
- If you bring your lunch to work, pack it in advance along with your healthy snacks for the day.
- Always try to account for contingencies by having some extra snacks available (e.g., energy bars, fruits, and measured-out nuts) for those occasions when you have to stay late at work, when you've skipped a meal to squeeze in a workout or worked through lunch, or any of a number of other things that can come up and throw you off your plan.

If you include your family in this task it can be a whole lot of fun, and very educational for them, too. Achieving goals as a family can be very rewarding.

Following are the abbreviations we will use in our five seven-day balanced calorie plans:

Nutrition Plan Key
C = Carbohydrates
P = Protein
F = Fat
Tbsp. = Tablespoon
Tspn. = Teaspoon
Oz. = Ounces
(e.g., 59 F = 59% fat)

Following are the five seven-day eating plans and the pages on which they begin:

- Plan 1500: 1,500 Balanced-Calorie Plan, page 161
- Plan 1750: 1,750 Balanced-Calorie Plan, page 168
- Plan 2000: 2,000 Balanced-Calorie Plan, page 175
- Plan 2250: 2,250 Balanced-Calorie Plan, page 182
- Plan 2500: 2,500 Balanced-Calorie Plan, page 189

Plan 1500: 1,500 Balanced-Calorie Seven-Day Eating Plan

DAY 1: 1500 Calorie Plan	Calorie Estimate

Note: Drink 8 oz. water with lemon/lime (0 Cal.) before all meals.

Breakfast:

Kashi flaxseed or blueberry waffles [Cal. %: 59 C, 11 P, 30 F]	150
Maple syrup—2 tbsp. [Cal. %: 99 C, 0 P, 1 F]	104
Egg—1, cooked with Pam [Cal. %: 2 C, 35 P, 63 F]	70
Coffee with skim milk	15
Total breakfast calories	**339**

Mid-Morning Snack:

Apple—1 small [Cal. %: 90 C, 0 P, 10 F]	55
Hard cheese—1 oz. [Cal. %: 2 C, 29 P, 69 F]	130
Total snack calories	**185**

Lunch:

Turkey breast—3 oz. [Cal. %: 0 C, 63 P, 37 F]	120
Rye bread—2 slices [Cal. %: 75 C, 14 P, 11 F]	130
Romaine lettuce—2 leaves [Cal. %: 75 C, 25 P, 0 F]	6
Mustard—2 tspn. [Cal. %: 42 C, 21 P, 37 F]	6
Baby carrots—4 [Cal. %: 90 C, 7 P, 3 F]	16
Total lunch calories	**278**

Midday Snack:

Strawberries—1 cup [Cal. %: 86 C, 6 P, 8 F]	45
Greek yogurt, 2%—4 oz. [Cal. %: 21 C, 52 P, 27 F]	80
Total snack calories	**125**

Dinner:

Flounder or sole—1 piece (6 oz.) [Cal. %: 1 C, 69 P, 30 F]	180
Baked potato—1 large [Cal. %: 74 C, 8 P, 18 F]	194
Butter—¹/₂ tbsp. [Cal. %: 0 C, 1 P, 99 F]	50
Mixed greens—1¹/₂ cups [Cal. %: 66 C, 26 P, 8 F]	15
Green beans, cooked—1 cup [Cal. %: 77 C, 20 P, 3 F]	34
Extra virgin olive oil—1 tbsp. [Cal. %: 0 C, 0 P, 100 F]	100
Total dinner calories	**573**

Total daily calories—Day 1	**1,500**

DAY 2: 1500 Calorie Plan	Calorie Estimate

Note: Drink 8 oz. water with lemon/lime (0 Cal.) before all meals.

Breakfast:

Cheerios—1 cup [Cal. %: 70 C, 12 P, 18 F]	100
Skim milk—1 cup [Cal. %: 54 C, 41 P, 5 F]	86
Blueberries—1 cup [Cal. %: 92 C, 3 P, 5 F]	83
Total breakfast calories	**269**

Mid-Morning Snack:

Brown rice cakes—2 [Cal. %: 87 C, 7 P, 6 F]	70
Organic creamy peanut butter—1½ tbsp. [Cal. %: 12 C, 16 P, 72 F]	150
Total snack calories	**220**

Lunch:

Tuna fish—3 oz. [Cal. %: 0 C, 63 P, 37 F]	168
Romaine lettuce—2 leaves [Cal. %: 75 C, 25 P, 0 F]	6
Light Caesar salad dressing—2 tbsp. [Cal. %: 11 C, 5 P, 84 F]	80
Apple—1 small [Cal. %: 90 C, 0 P, 10 F]	55
Total lunch calories	**309**

Midday Snack:

ZonePerfect Bar [Cal. %: 47 C, 21 P, 32 F]	200
Total snack calories	**200**

Dinner:

Chicken sausage—2 links [Cal. %: 6 C, 46 P, 48 F]	260
Whole-grain brown rice—³/₄ cup [Cal. %: 84 C, 10 P, 6 F]	112
Steamed broccoli with lemon—³/₄ cup [Cal. %: 66 C, 25 P, 9 F]	30
Total dinner calories	**402**

Evening Snack:

Smartfood white cheddar popcorn [Cal. %: 37 C, 8 P, 55 F]	100
Total snack calories	**100**

Total daily calories—Day 2	**1,500**

DAY 3: 1500 Calorie Plan	Calorie Estimate

Note: Drink 8 oz. water with lemon/lime (0 Cal.) before all meals.

Breakfast:

Steel-cut oatmeal—1/4 cup [Cal. %: 72 C, 13 P, 15 F]	150
Brown sugar—1 tspn. [Cal. %: 100 C, 0 P, 0 F]	15
Walnuts, chopped—$^1/_8$ cup [Cal. %: 8 C, 8 P, 84 F]	100
Peach—1 medium [Cal. %: 87 C, 8 P, 5 F]	38
Total breakfast calories	**303**

Mid-Morning Snack:

Cottage cheese, 2%—4 oz. or $^1/_2$ cup [Cal. %: 16 C, 65 P, 19 F]	100
Pineapple—2 slices, $^3/_4$-inch-thick [Cal. %: 95 C, 3 P, 2 F]	80
Total snack calories	**180**

Lunch:

Turkey burger (3 oz.), lettuce, and tomato [Cal. %: 10 C, 35 P, 55 F]	200
Whole-wheat pita—medium [Cal. %: 80 C, 15 P, 5 F]	123
Ketchup—1 tbsp. [Cal. %: 100 C, 0 P, 0 F]	20
Baby carrots—6 [Cal. %: 90 C, 7 P, 3 F]	24
Total lunch calories	**367**

Midday Snack:

Pear [Cal. %: 96 C, 2 P, 2 F]	96
Mozzarella stick [Cal. %: 5 C, 35 P, 60 F]	85
Total snack calories	**181**

Dinner:

Whole-wheat spaghetti—1 cup [Cal. %: 81 C, 15 P, 4 F]	185
Chicken (or vegetable) broth—1 cup [Cal. %: 50 C, 28 P, 22 F]	12
Chickpeas—$^1/_2$ cup [Cal. %: 67 C, 20 P, 13 F]	100
Shrimp—6 [Cal. %: 0 C, 100 P, 0 F]	70
Fresh parsley—1 cup, chopped [Cal. %: 63 C, 19 P, 18 F]	22
Total dinner calories	**389**

Evening Snack:

Skim milk—8 oz. [Cal. %: 51 C, 44 P, 5 F]	80
Total snack calories	**80**

Total daily calories—Day 3	**1,500**

DAY 4: 1500 Calorie Plan	Calorie Estimate

Note: Drink 8 oz. water with lemon/lime (0 Cal.) before all meals.

Breakfast:

Oat-bran English muffin—1 [Cal. %: 72 C, 15 P, 13 F]	125
Egg—1 large scrambled, cooked with Pam [Cal. %: 5 C, 29 P, 66 F]	101
Grapefruit—$1/2$ [Cal. %: 91 C, 6 P, 3 F]	52
Total breakfast calories	**278**

Mid-Morning Snack:

Carrots, celery, tomatoes, peppers—$1^1/2$ cups [Cal. %: 82 C, 10 P, 8 F]	100
Reduced-fat ranch dressing—2 tbsp. [Cal. %: 28 C, 2 P, 70 F]	70
Total snack calories	**170**

Lunch:

Grilled chicken breast—3 oz. [Cal. %: 0 C, 63 P, 37 F]	165
Low-fat cheddar cheese—1 slice [Cal. %: 0 C, 44 P, 56 F]	70
Romaine lettuce—4 leaves [Cal. %: 75 C, 25 P, 0 F]	12
Organic blue corn chips—6 chips [Cal. %: 55 C, 6 P, 39 F]	140
Baby carrots—6 [Cal. %: 90 C, 7 P, 3 F]	24
Total lunch calories	**411**

Midday Snack:

Apple—1 medium [Cal. %: 90 C, 0 P, 10 F]	80
Total snack calories	**80**

Dinner:

Split-pea soup—1 cup [Cal. %: 64 C, 20 P, 16 F]	165
Croutons—$3/4$ cup [Cal. %: 55 C, 9 P, 36 F]	140
Mozzarella cheese, partial skim—2 sticks [Cal. %: 5 C, 35 P, 60 F]	170
Total dinner calories	**475**

Evening Snack:

Applesauce, unsweetened—$3/4$ cup [Cal. %: 98 C, 1 P, 1 F]	86
Total snack calories	**86**

Total daily calories—Day 4	**1,500**

DAY 5: 1500 Calorie Plan	Calorie Estimate

Note: Drink 8 oz. water with lemon/lime (0 Cal.) before all meals.

Breakfast:

French toast—2 slices [Cal. %: 60 C, 15 P, 25 F]	252
Butter—¹/₃ tbsp. [Cal. %: 0 C, 1 P, 99 F]	36
Vegetable juice—¹/₂ cup [Cal. %: 75 C, 18 P, 7 F]	36
Total breakfast calories	**324**

Mid-Morning Snack:

Greek yogurt, 2%, with fruit—1 cup or 8 oz. [Cal. %: 22 C, 54 P, 24 F]	140
Total snack calories	**140**

Lunch:

Egg-white and chive salad with light mayo—6 oz. [Cal. %: 15 C, 52 P, 33 F]	100
Rye bread—2 slices [Cal. %: 75 C, 14 P, 11 F]	130
Romaine lettuce—2 leaves [Cal. %: 75 C, 25 P, 0 F]	6
Cantaloupe—1 cup [Cal. %: 86 C, 9 P, 5 F]	60
Blueberries—¹/₂ cup [Cal. %: 92 C, 3 P, 5 F]	42
Total lunch calories	**338**

Midday Snack:

Whole almonds—¹/₄ cup [Cal. %: 14 C, 13 P, 73 F]	170
Dried fig—1 [Cal. %: 14 C, 13 P, 73 F]	42
Total snack calories	**212**

Dinner:

Lasagna with meat—1 piece (3 x 4 in.) [Cal. %: 42 C, 25 P, 33 F]	336
Mixed green salad—1¹/₂ cups [Cal. %: 66 C, 26 P, 8 F]	15
Olive oil dressing—¹/₂ tbsp. and lemon juice—1 tbsp. [Cal. %: 2 C, 0 P, 98 F]	66
Total dinner calories	**417**

Evening Snack:

Navel orange [Cal. %: 92 C, 5 P, 3 F]	69
Total snack calories	**69**

Total daily calories—Day 5	**1,500**

DAY 6: 1500 Calorie Plan	Calorie Estimate

Note: Drink 8 oz. water with lemon/lime (0 Cal.) before all meals.

Breakfast:

Soy protein shake—1 scoop [Cal. %: 51 C, 42 P, 7 F]	130
Plain yogurt, 1%—³/₄ cup [Cal. %: 45 C, 33 P, 22 F]	105
Mixed berries, frozen or fresh—1 cup [Cal. %: 94 C, 6 P, 0 F]	70
Total breakfast calories	**305**

Mid-Morning Snack:

Rye bread—1 slice [Cal. %: 75 C, 14 P, 11 F]	65
Organic almond or peanut butter—1 tbsp. [Cal. %: 12 C, 16 P, 72 F]	100
Total snack calories	**165**

Lunch:

Turkey breast—3 oz. [Cal. %: 15 C, 52 P, 33 F]	120
Cheddar cheese, 2%—2 slices [Cal. %: 0 C, 44 P, 56 F]	140
Romaine lettuce—2 leaves [Cal. %: 75 C, 25 P, 0 F]	6
Apple—1 medium [Cal. %: 90 C, 0 P, 10 F]	80
Total lunch calories	**346**

Midday Snack:

Pear—1 medium [Cal. %: 96 C, 2 P, 2 F]	96
Cheese stick (light) [Cal. %: 0 C, 44 P, 56 F]	45
Total snack calories	**141**

Dinner:

Rotisserie chicken—4 oz. [Cal. %: 0 C, 47 P, 53 F]	150
Sweet potato—1 medium [Cal. %: 94 C, 6 P, 0 F]	112
Butter (for sweet potato)—1 tbsp. [Cal. %: 0 C, 1 P, 99 F]	100
Mixed green salad—1¹/₂ cups [Cal. %: 66 C, 26 P, 8 F]	15
Olive oil dressing—¹/₂ tbsp. and lemon—1 tbsp. [Cal. %: 2 C, 0 P, 98 F]	66
Total dinner calories	**443**

Evening Snack:

Dark chocolate–covered almonds—6 pieces [Cal. %: 43 C, 4 P, 53 F]	100
Total snack calories	**100**

Total daily calories—Day 6	**1,500**

DAY 7: 1500 Calorie Plan	Calorie Estimate

Note: Drink 8 oz. water with lemon/lime (0 Cal.) before all meals.

Breakfast:

Omelet—2 medium eggs, cooked with Pam [Cal. %: 2 C, 35 P, 63 F]	150
Chopped potato, medium, browned in Pam [Cal. %: 91 C, 8 P, 1 F]	121
Cheddar cheese, 2%—1 slice [Cal. %: 0 C, 44 P, 56 F]	70
Total breakfast calories	**341**

Mid-Morning Snack:

Whole almonds—20 [Cal. %: 14 C, 13 P, 73 F]	140
Total snack calories	**140**

Lunch:

California sushi roll—4 pieces [Cal. %: 67 C, 11 P, 22 F]	300
Miso soup—1 cup [Cal. %: 36 C, 29 P, 35 F]	84
Total lunch calories	**384**

Midday Snack:

Apple—1 medium [Cal. %: 90 C, 0 P, 10 F]	80
Organic peanut butter—1 tbsp. [Cal. %: 12 C, 16 P, 72 F]	100
Total snack calories	**180**

Dinner:

Whole-wheat pasta—1 cup [Cal. %: 80 C, 16 P, 4 F]	170
Sun-dried tomatoes—3 pieces [Cal. %: 43 C, 9 P, 48 F]	45
Broccoli—1 cup, cooked [Cal. %: 70 C, 21 P, 9 F]	31
Extra virgin olive oil—1 tbsp. [Cal. %: 0 C, 0 P, 100 F]	100
Italian bread—1 medium piece [Cal. %: 76 C, 13 P, 11 F]	54
Total dinner calories	**400**

Evening Snack:

Graham cracker—1 [Cal. %: 73 C, 6 P, 21 F]	55
Total snack calories	**55**

Total daily calories—Day 7	**1,500**

Plan 1750: 1,750 Balanced-Calorie Seven-Day Eating Plan

DAY 1: 1750 Calorie Plan	Calorie Estimate

Note: Drink 8 oz. water with lemon/lime (0 Cal.) before all meals.

Breakfast:

Quick-cook oatmeal—½ cup [Cal. %: 72 C, 13 P, 15 F]	150
Blueberries—½ cup [Cal. %: 92 C, 3 P, 5 F]	42
Hard-boiled egg—1 large [Cal. %: 3 C, 33 P, 64 F]	75
Grapefruit juice—1 cup [Cal. %: 92 C, 6 P, 2 F]	96
Total breakfast calories	**363**

Mid-Morning Snack:

Baked Whole SOYJOY Bar [Cal. %: 52 C, 12 P, 36 F]	140
Total snack calories	**140**

Lunch:

Grilled chicken breast—3 oz. [Cal. %: 0 C, 63 P, 37 F]	165
Spinach wrap, small—2 oz. [Cal. %: 36 C, 29 P, 35 F]	160
Cheddar cheese, 2%—1 slice [Cal. %: 0 C, 44 P, 56 F]	70
Romaine lettuce—4 leaves [Cal. %: 75 C, 25 P, 0 F]	12
Light mayo—2 tbsp. [Cal. %: 15 C, 0 P, 85 F]	70
Total lunch calories	**477**

Midday Snack:

Whole almonds—18 [Cal. %: 14 C, 13 P, 73 F]	126
Plain nonfat yogurt—1 cup [Cal. %: 54 C, 46 P, 0 F]	130
Total snack calories	**256**

Dinner:

Whole-wheat pasta—1 cup [Cal. %: 80 C, 16 P, 4 F]	170
Broccoli—1 cup, cooked [Cal. %: 70 C, 21 P, 9 F]	30
Diced tomatoes—1 cup [Cal. %: 86 C, 14 P, 0 F]	60
Extra virgin olive oil—1 tbsp. [Cal. %: 0 C, 0 P, 100 F]	100
Grated Parmesan cheese—1 tbsp. [Cal. %: 0 C, 37 P, 63 F]	20
Italian bread—1 medium piece [Cal. %: 76 C, 13 P, 11 F]	54
Total dinner calories	**434**

Evening Snack:

Apple—1 medium [Cal. %: 90 C, 0 P, 10 F]	80
Total snack calories	**80**

Total daily calories—Day 1	**1,750**

DAY 2: 1750 Calorie Plan	Calorie Estimate

Note: Drink 8 oz. water with lemon/lime (0 Cal.) before all meals.

Breakfast:

Cheerios, plain—1 cup [Cal. %: 72 C, 13 P, 15 F]	100
Banana, medium [Cal. %: 92 C, 5 P, 3 F]	105
Skim milk—1 cup [Cal. %: 54 C, 41 P, 5 F]	86
Sliced almonds—1/8 cup [Cal. %: 14 C, 13 P, 73 F]	67
Total breakfast calories	**358**

Mid-Morning Snack:

Cottage cheese, 2%—3/4 cup [Cal. %: 25 C, 51 P, 24 F]	150
Pineapple—1 slice [Cal. %: 95 C, 3 P, 2 F]	40
Total snack calories	**190**

Lunch:

Vegetable soup—2 cups [Cal. %: 93 C, 7 P, 0 F]	120
Corn tortilla—1 round [Cal. %: 82 C, 7 P, 11 F]	60
Avocado—1 medium [Cal. %: 19 C, 4 P, 77 F]	322
Total lunch calories	**502**

Midday Snack:

Greek yogurt, 2% with fruit—1 cup or 8 oz. [Cal. %: 22 C, 54 P, 24 F]	140
Total snack calories	**140**

Dinner:

Turkey meatloaf—1 large slice (4 oz.) [Cal. %: 18 C, 49 P, 33 F]	220
Baked potato—1 large [Cal. %: 74 C, 8 P, 18 F]	195
Mixed green salad—1 cup [Cal. %: 66 C, 26 P, 8 F]	10
Olive oil dressing—1/2 tbsp. and lemon juice—1 tbsp. [Cal. %: 2 C, 0 P, 98 F]	66
Total dinner calories	**491**

Evening Snack:

Navel orange [Cal. %: 92 C, 5 P, 3 F]	69
Total snack calories	**69**

| **Total daily calories—Day 2** | **1,750** |

DAY 3: 1750 Calorie Plan	Calorie Estimate

Note: Drink 8 oz. water with lemon/lime (0 Cal.) before all meals.

Breakfast:

Rye bread—2 slices [Cal. %: 75 C, 13 P, 12 F]	134
Butter—1 tbsp. [Cal. %: 0 C, 1P, 99F]	102
Orange juice—6 oz. [Cal. %: 95 C, 5 P, 0 F]	112
Total breakfast calories	**348**

Mid-Morning Snack:

Fruit and nut trail mix—3 tbsp. [Cal. %: 36 C, 8 P, 56 F]	140
Pear [Cal. %: 96 C, 2 P, 2 F]	96
Total snack calories	**236**

Lunch:

Tuna fish—5 oz., and 2 lettuce leaves [Cal. %: 18 C, 80 P, 2 F]	263
Light mayo—2 tbsp. [Cal. %: 15 C, 0 P, 85 F]	70
Multigrain brown rice cakes—3 [Cal. %: 85 C, 7 P, 8 F]	105
Baby carrots—4 [Cal. %: 90 C, 7 P, 3 F]	16
Total lunch calories	**454**

Midday Snack:

Celery stalks—3 [Cal. %: 76 C, 14 P, 10 F]	18
Organic peanut butter—1½ tbsp. [Cal. %: 12 C, 16 P, 72 F]	150
Total snack calories	**168**

Dinner:

Roasted white-meat chicken—3 oz. [Cal. %: 0 C, 38 P, 62 F]	160
Sweet potato [Cal. %: 94 C, 6 P, 0 F]	112
Butter (for sweet potato)—1 tbsp. [Cal. %: 0 C, 1 P, 99 F]	102
Boston lettuce, 1 cup, with lite dressing—1 tbsp. [Cal. %: 55 C, 33 P, 12 F]	65
Brussels sprouts, steamed with lemon—1 cup [Cal. %: 74 C, 20 P, 6 F]	38
Total dinner calories	**477**

Evening Snack:

Dark chocolate–covered almonds—4 pieces [Cal. %: 43 C, 4 P, 53 F]	67
Total snack calories	**67**

| **Total daily calories—Day 3** | **1,750** |

DAY 4: 1750 Calorie Plan   Calorie Estimate

Note: Drink 8 oz. water with lemon/lime (0 Cal.) before all meals.

Breakfast:

Omelet—2 medium eggs, cooked with Pam [Cal. %: 2 C, 35 P, 63 F]	150
Tomato—1 medium [Cal. %: 75 C, 16 P, 9 F]	24
Feta cheese—1/4 cup [Cal. %: 7 C, 40 P, 53 F]	75
Grapefruit juice—6 oz. [Cal. %: 95 C, 5 P, 0 F]	75
Total breakfast calories	**324**

Mid-Morning Snack:

Apple—1 medium [Cal. %: 90 C, 0 P, 10 F]	80
Cheese sticks, light—2 [Cal. %: 0 C, 44 P, 56 F]	90
Total snack calories	**170**

Lunch:

Turkey breast—5 oz. [Cal. %: 0 C, 63 P, 37 F]	200
Rye bread—2 slices [Cal. %: 75 C, 14 P, 11 F]	130
Romaine lettuce—2 leaves [Cal. %: 75 C, 25 P, 0 F]	6
Low-fat cheddar cheese—1 slice [Cal. %: 0 C, 44 P, 56 F]	70
Mustard—2 tspn. [Cal. %: 42 C, 21 P, 37 F]	6
Baby carrots—5 [Cal. %: 90 C, 7 P, 3 F]	16
Total lunch calories	**428**

Midday Snack:

Unsweetened applesauce—1 1/2 cups [Cal. %: 90 C, 0 P, 10 F]	75
Sliced almonds—1/8 cup [Cal. %: 14 C, 13 P, 73 F]	134
Total snack calories	**209**

Dinner:

Lasagna with ground beef or turkey—1 piece (3.5 x 4 in.) [Cal. %: 42 C, 25 P, 33 F]	378
Mixed green salad—1 1/2 cups [Cal. %: 66 C, 26 P, 8 F]	15
Olive oil / balsamic vinegar dressing—1/2 tbsp. [Cal. %: 2 C, 0 P, 98 F]	66
Asparagus—8 large spears [Cal. %: 36 C, 20 P, 44 F]	64
Total dinner calories	**523**

Evening Snack:

Pear [Cal. %: 96 C, 2 P, 2 F]	96
Total snack calories	**96**
Total daily calories—Day 4	**1,750**

DAY 5: 1750 Calorie Plan	Calorie Estimate

Note: Drink 8 oz. water with lemon/lime (0 Cal.) before all meals.

Breakfast:

Greek yogurt, 2%, plain—1 cup or 8 oz. [Cal. %: 22 C, 54 P, 24 F]	140
Low-fat granola—1/2 cup [Cal. %: 80 C, 8 P, 12 F]	210
Grapefruit juice—6 oz. [Cal. %: 95 C, 5 P, 0 F]	75
Total breakfast calories	**425**

Mid-Morning Snack:

ZonePerfect Bar [Cal. %: 41 C, 29 P, 30 F]	200
Total snack calories	**200**

Lunch:

Split-pea soup—1 1/2 cups [Cal. %: 64 C, 20 P, 16 F]	248
Smoked honey ham, sliced—3 oz. [Cal. %: 24 C, 59 P, 17 F]	107
Whole-wheat pita, medium—1 [Cal. %: 80 C, 15 P, 5 F]	123
Romaine lettuce—3 leaves [Cal. %: 75 C, 25 P, 0 F]	9
Mustard—2 tspn. [Cal. %: 42 C, 21 P, 37 F]	7
Total lunch calories	**494**

Midday Snack:

Pear [Cal. %: 96 C, 2 P, 2 F]	96
Mozzarella stick—1 [Cal. %: 5 C, 35 P, 60 F]	85
Total snack calories	**181**

Dinner:

Spinach tortellini—1 cup [Cal. %: 81 C, 15 P, 4 F]	229
Chicken (or vegetable) broth—1 cup [Cal. %: 50 C, 28 P, 22 F]	12
Italian bread—1 slice [Cal. %: 76 C, 13 P, 11 F]	108
Fresh parsley, chopped—1 cup [Cal. %: 63 C, 19 P, 18 F]	21
Total dinner calories	**370**

Evening Snack:

Skim milk—8 oz. [Cal. %: 51 C, 44 P, 5 F]	80
Total snack calories	**80**
Total daily calories—Day 5	**1,750**

DAY 6: 1750 Calorie Plan	Calorie Estimate

Note: Drink 8 oz. water with lemon/lime (0 Cal.) before all meals.

Breakfast:

Cottage cheese, 2%—1 cup or 8 oz. [Cal. %: 16 C, 65 P, 19 F]	200
Cantaloupe—1½ cups [Cal. %: 86 C, 9 P, 5 F]	85
Blueberries—½ cup [Cal. %: 92 C, 3 P, 5 F]	42
Total breakfast calories	**327**

Mid-Morning Snack:

Whole almonds—20 [Cal. %: 14 C, 13 P, 73 F]	140
Grapes, seedless—½ cup [Cal. %: 94 C, 4 P, 2 F]	55
Total snack calories	**195**

Lunch:

Lean beef or turkey burger—4 oz. [Cal. %: 4 C, 69 P, 27 F]	160
Spinach wrap, small—2 oz. [Cal. %: 36 C, 29 P, 35 F]	160
Cheddar cheese, 2%—1 slice [Cal. %: 0 C, 44 P, 56 F]	70
Field greens [Cal. %: 80 C, 20 P, 0 F]	25
Baked lentil chips—11 chips [Cal. %: 64 C, 13 P, 23 F]	55
Total lunch calories	**470**

Midday Snack:

Hard-boiled eggs, large—2 [Cal. %: 3 C, 33 P, 64 F]	157
Total snack calories	**157**

Dinner:

Chicken sausage—1 link, or 3 oz. [Cal. %: 4 C, 42 P, 54 F]	140
Whole-wheat pasta—1 cup [Cal. %: 80 C, 16 P, 4 F]	170
Diced cooked tomatoes—1 cup [Cal. %: 86 C, 14 P, 0 F]	60
Broccoli, cooked—1 cup [Cal. %: 70 C, 21 P, 9 F]	31
Extra virgin olive oil—1 tbsp. [Cal. %: 0 C, 0 P, 100 F]	100
Total dinner calories	**501**

Evening Snack:

Smartfood white cheddar popcorn [Cal. %: 37 C, 8 P, 55 F]	100
Total snack calories	**100**

Total daily calories—Day 6	**1,750**

DAY 7: 1750 Calorie Plan	Calorie Estimate

Note: Drink 8 oz. water with lemon/lime (0 Cal.) before all meals.

Breakfast:

Bonk Breaker Energy Bar [Cal. %: 76 C, 13 P, 11 F]	220
Cappuccino with skim milk [Cal. %: 39 C, 27 P, 34 F]	90
Total breakfast calories	**310**

Mid-Morning Snack:

Goat cheese, hard—1 oz. [Cal. %: 2 C, 29 P, 69 F]	128
Whole-grain pita chips—7 chips [Cal. %: 57 C, 9 P, 34 F]	70
Red grapes, seedless—1/2 cup [Cal. %: 94 C, 4 P, 2 F]	55
Total snack calories	**253**

Lunch:

Egg-white salad with light mayo and lettuce—6 oz. [Cal. %: 19 C, 45 P, 36 F]	184
Whole-wheat pita, medium—1 [Cal. %: 80 C, 15 P, 5 F]	123
Baby carrots—6 [Cal. %: 90 C, 7 P, 3 F]	24
Apple—1 medium [Cal. %: 90 C, 0 P, 10 F]	80
Total lunch calories	**411**

Midday Snack:

Banana, large—1 [Cal. %: 92 C, 5 P, 3 F]	110
Whole almonds—15 [Cal. %: 14 C, 14 P, 72 F]	105
Total snack calories	**215**

Dinner:

Lentil soup—1 1/2 cups [Cal. %: 18 C, 22 P, 60 F]	270
Wasa Whole-Grain Crispbread—3 crackers [Cal. %: 91 C, 9 P, 0 F]	120
Laughing Cow Swiss cheese—2 wedges [Cal. %: 16 C, 31 P, 53 F]	70
Total dinner calories	**460**

Evening Snack:

Fat-free chocolate pudding cup [Cal. %: 84 C, 12 P, 4 F]	101
Total snack calories	**101**

Total daily calories—Day 7	1,750

Plan 2000: 2,000 Balanced-Calorie Seven-Day Eating Plan

DAY 1: 2000 Calorie Plan	Calorie Estimate

Note: Drink 8 oz. water with lemon/lime (0 Cal.) before all meals.

Breakfast:

Multigrain English muffin—1 [Cal. %: 71 C, 13 P, 16 F]	150
Organic creamy peanut butter—2 tbsp. [Cal. %:12 C, 16 P, 72 F]	200
Raspberry preserves—¹/₂ tbsp. [Cal. %: 100 C, 0 P, 0 F]	25
Total breakfast calories	**375**

Mid-Morning Snack:

Vegetable juice, V8 low-sodium—8 oz. [Cal. %: 83 C, 17 P, 0 F]	50
Wasa Light Rye Crispbread—2 crackers [Cal. %: 91 C, 9 P, 0 F]	60
Light string cheese—2 sticks [Cal. %: 8 C, 47 P, 45 F]	100
Hummus—2 tbsp. [Cal. %: 45 C, 11 P, 44 F]	54
Total snack calories	**264**

Lunch:

Bumble Bee Tuna Medley, Lemon Pepper—6 oz. [Cal. %: 7 C, 68 P, 25 F]	220
Rye bread—2 slices [Cal. %: 75 C, 14 P, 11 F]	130
Light mayo—2 tbsp. [Cal. %: 15 C, 0 P, 85 F]	70
Baby spinach—1 cup [Cal. %: 49 C, 39 P, 12 F]	7
Total lunch calories	**427**

Midday Snack:

Clif Mojo Bar [Cal. %: 30 C, 16 P, 55 F]	200
Skim milk—1 cup [Cal. %: 54 C, 41 P, 5 F]	86
Total snack calories	**286**

Dinner:

Lean turkey chili with beans—1¹/₂ cups [Cal. %: 36 C, 34 P, 30 F]	332
Cheddar cheese, 2%, on top—1 slice [Cal. %: 4 C, 24 P, 72 F]	45
Tostitos blue corn chips—6 big chips [Cal. %: 55 C, 6 P, 39 F]	140
Total dinner calories	**517**

Evening Snack:

Pear [Cal. %: 96 C, 2 P, 2 F]	96
Laughing Cow Swiss cheese—1 wedge [Cal. %: 16 C, 31 P, 53 F]	35
Total snack calories	**131**

Total daily calories—Day 1	**2,000**

DAY 2: 2000 Calorie Plan	Calorie Estimate

Note: Drink 8 oz. water with lemon/lime (0 Cal.) before all meals.

Breakfast

Steel-cut oatmeal—$^1/_4$ cup [Cal. %: 72 C, 13 P, 15 F]	150
Blueberries—1 cup [Cal. %: 92 C, 3 P, 5 F]	84
Walnuts, chopped—$^1/_8$ cup [Cal. %: 8 C, 8 P, 84 F]	100
Brown sugar—$3^1/_2$ tspn. [Cal. %: 100 C, 0 P, 0 F]	53
Total breakfast calories	**387**

Mid-Morning Snack:

Laughing Cow Swiss cheese—2 wedges [Cal. %: 16 C, 31 P, 53 F]	70
Wasa Whole-Grain Crispbread—2 crackers [Cal. %: 91 C, 9 P, 0 F]	80
Apple—1 medium [Cal. %: 90 C, 0 P, 10 F]	80
Total snack calories	**230**

Lunch:

Boca Burger, flame-grilled [Cal. %: 19 C, 45 P, 36 F]	120
Mixed greens—$1^1/_2$ cups [Cal. %: 66 C, 26 P, 8 F]	12
Crumbled Gorgonzola cheese—$^1/_4$ cup [Cal. %: 4 C, 24 P, 72 F]	100
Cranraisins—$^1/_3$ cup [Cal. %: 100 C, 0 P, 0 F]	140
Sunflower seeds, shelled—$^1/_8$ cup [Cal. %: 11 C, 19 P, 71 F]	95
Total lunch calories	**467**

Midday Snack:

Kashi Dark Mocha Almond Bar [Cal. %: 43 C, 4 P, 53 F]	130
Banana, large—1 [Cal. %: 92 C, 5 P, 3 F]	110
Total snack calories	**240**

Dinner:

Potato-crusted fish fillets—3 (3.4 oz.) [Cal. %: 18 C, 22 P, 60 F]	403
Whole-grain brown rice—$^3/_4$ cup [Cal. %: 84 C, 10 P, 6 F]	112
Steamed broccoli with lemon [Cal. %: 66 C, 25 P, 9 F]	41
Total dinner calories	**556**

Evening Snack:

Light popcorn—$3^1/_2$ cups [Cal. %: 96 C, 2 P, 2 F]	120
Total snack calories	**120**

Total daily calories—Day 2	**2,000**

DAY 3: 2000 Calorie Plan	Calorie Estimate

Note: Drink 8 oz. water with lemon/lime (0 Cal.) before all meals.

Breakfast:

Bonk Breaker Energy Bar [Cal. %: 76 C, 13 P, 11 F]	225
Cappuccino with skim milk [Cal. %: 39 C, 27 P, 34 F]	90
Total breakfast calories	**315**

Mid-Morning Snack:

Goat cheese, hard—1 oz. [Cal. %: 2 C, 29 P, 69 F]	128
Reduced-fat Triscuits—4 crackers [Cal. %: 18 F, 73 C, 9 P]	69
Red grapes, seedless—1/2 cup [Cal. %: 94 C, 4 P, 2 F]	55
Total snack calories	**252**

Lunch:

Egg-white salad with light mayo—6 oz. [Cal. %: 19 C, 45 P, 36 F]	184
Rye bread—2 slices [Cal. %: 75 C, 14 P, 11 F]	130
Romaine lettuce—2 leaves [Cal. %: 75 C, 25 P, 0 F]	6
Baby carrots—6 [Cal. %: 90 C, 7 P, 3 F]	24
Applesauce, unsweetened—1 cup [Cal. %: 90 C, 0 P, 10 F]	50
Total lunch calories	**394**

Midday Snack:

Pineapple—2 slices, 3/4-inch thick [Cal. %: 95 C, 3 P, 2 F]	80
Cottage cheese, 2%—1 cup or 8 oz. [Cal. %: 16 C, 65 P, 19 F]	200
Total snack calories	**280**

Dinner:

Chicken and wild rice soup—2 cups [Cal. %: 62 C, 24 P, 14 F]	200
French roll [Cal. %: 74 C, 12 P, 14 F]	105
Butter (for French roll)—1 tbsp. [Cal. %: 0 C, 1 P, 99 F]	102
Mixed green salad—1 1/2 cups [Cal. %: 66 C, 26 P, 8 F]	15
Feta cheese—1/4 cup [Cal. %: 7 C, 40 P, 53 F]	75
Olive oil / vinegar dressing—1/2 tbsp. [Cal. %: 2 C, 0 P, 98 F]	66
Total dinner calories	**563**

Evening Snack:

Dark chocolate peanut butter cups—4 pieces [Cal. %: 96 C, 2 P, 2 F]	196
Total snack calories	**196**

| **Total daily calories—Day 3** | **2,000** |

DAY 4: 2000 Calorie Plan	Calorie Estimate

Note: Drink 8 oz. water with lemon/lime (0 Cal.) before all meals.

Breakfast:

Light-style seven-grain bread, toasted—2 slices [Cal. %: 71 C, 22 P, 7 F]	90
Light cream cheese—1 tbsp. [Cal. %: 15 C, 16 P, 69 F]	30
Omelet—2 medium eggs, cooked with Pam [Cal. %: 2 C, 35 P, 63 F]	150
Grapefruit juice—6 oz. [Cal. %: 95 C, 5 P, 0 F]	75
Total breakfast calories	**345**

Mid-Morning Snack:

Fruit and nut trail mix—3 tbsp. [Cal. %: 36 C, 8 P, 56 F]	140
Peaches in light syrup—1 cup [Cal. %: 87 C, 8 P, 5 F]	138
Total snack calories	**278**

Lunch:

Tuna fish, 5 oz., and 2 leaves of lettuce [Cal. %: 18 C, 80 P, 2 F]	114
Cheddar cheese, 2%—2 slices [Cal. %: 4 C, 24 P, 72 F]	90
Light mayo—2 tbsp. [Cal. %: 15 C, 0 P, 85 F]	70
Multigrain brown rice cakes—2 [Cal. %: 85 C, 7 P, 8 F]	70
Baby carrots—6 [Cal. %: 90 C, 7 P, 3 F]	24
Total lunch calories	**368**

Midday Snack:

Apple—1 medium [Cal. %: 90 C, 0 P, 10 F]	80
Organic peanut butter—2 tbsp. [Cal. %: 12 C, 16 P, 72 F]	200
Total snack calories	**280**

Dinner:

Roasted white-meat chicken—5 oz. [Cal. %: 0 C, 38 P, 62 F]	266
Sweet potato [Cal. %: 94 C, 6 P, 0 F]	112
Butter (for sweet potato)—1 tbsp. [Cal. %: 0 C, 1 P, 99 F]	102
Boston lettuce (1 cup) with lite dressing (1 tbsp.) [Cal. %: 55 C, 33 P, 12 F]	65
Brussels sprouts, steamed with lemon—1 cup [Cal. %: 74 C, 20 P, 6 F]	38
Total dinner calories	**583**

Evening Snack:

Strawberries—1 cup [Cal. %: 86 C, 6 P, 8 F]	46
Greek yogurt, 2%—5 oz. [Cal. %: 21 C, 52 P, 27 F]	100
Total snack calories	**146**

| **Total daily calories—Day 4** | **2,000** |

DAY 5: 2000 Calorie Plan   Calorie Estimate

Note: Drink 8 oz. water with lemon/lime (0 Cal.) before all meals.

Breakfast:

Spinach omelet—2 large eggs, cooked with Pam [Cal. %: 2 C, 35 P, 63 F]	154
Multigrain English muffin, regular—1 [Cal. %: 71 C, 13 P, 16 F]	150
Reduced-sugar raspberry jelly—2 tbsp. [Cal. %: 100 C, 0 P, 0 F]	70
Total breakfast calories	**374**

Mid-Morning Snack:

Banana, medium—1 [Cal. %: 92 C, 5 P, 3 F]	105
Almond butter—1 tbsp. [Cal. %: 13 C, 8 P, 79 F]	200
Total snack calories	**305**

Lunch:

Chicken salad with celery and carrots—5 oz. [Cal. %: 0 C, 63 P, 37 F]	250
Light mayo—2 tbsp. [Cal. %: 15 C, 0 P, 85 F]	70
Simply Naked Pita Chips—1 oz. (or about 10 chips) [Cal. %: 55 C, 10 P, 35 F]	130
Total lunch calories	**450**

Midday Snack:

Clif Bar [Cal. %: 68 C, 15 P, 17 F]	240
Total snack calories	**240**

Dinner:

Eggplant, cooked—6 slices [Cal. %: 47 C, 4 P, 49 F]	213
Light mozzarella cheese—1.5 oz. [Cal. %: 0 C, 43 P, 57 F]	68
Tomato sauce—1 cup [Cal. %: 70 C, 14 P, 16 F]	120
Italian bread—1 medium piece [Cal. %: 76 C, 13 P, 11 F]	54
Asparagus, fresh, steamed—6 spears [Cal. %: 36 C, 20 P, 44 F]	30
Total dinner calories	**485**

Evening Snack:

Strawberries—1 cup [Cal. %: 86 C, 6 P, 8 F]	46
Greek yogurt, 2%—5 oz. [Cal. %: 21 C, 52 P, 27 F]	100
Total snack calories	**146**

Total daily calories—Day 5	**2,000**

DAY 6: 2000 Calorie Plan	Calorie Estimate

Note: Drink 8 oz. water with lemon/lime (0 Cal.) before all meals.

Breakfast:

Cottage cheese, 2%—1 cup or 8 oz. [Cal. %: 16 C, 65 P, 19 F]	200
Cantaloupe—1 cup [Cal. %: 86 C, 9 P, 5 F]	60
Blueberries—1 cup [Cal. %: 92 C, 3 P, 5 F]	84
Total breakfast calories	**344**

Mid-Morning Snack:

Apple—1 medium [Cal. %: 90 C, 0 P, 10 F]	80
Pistachios—½ cup with shells [Cal. %: 10 C, 15 P, 75 F]	160
Total snack calories	**240**

Lunch:

Grilled chicken breast—4 oz. [Cal. %: 0 C, 63 P, 37 F]	208
Field greens or spinach—2 cups [Cal. %: 61 C, 29 P, 10 F]	18
Red peppers, celery, onions, mushrooms, raw—1 cup [Cal. %: 98 C, 2 P, 0 F]	50
Feta cheese—¼ cup [Cal. %: 7 C, 40 P, 53 F]	75
Smartfood white cheddar popcorn [Cal. %: 37 C, 8 P, 55 F]	100
Total lunch calories	**451**

Midday Snack:

Organic peanut butter—2 tbsp. [Cal. %: 12 C, 16 P, 72 F]	200
Celery sticks—4 [Cal. %: 76 C, 14 P, 10 F]	24
Total snack calories	**224**

Dinner:

Hearty black bean soup—1½ cups [Cal. %: 7 C, 19 P, 8 F]	255
Light mozzarella cheese—1 oz. [Cal. %: 0 C, 43 P, 57 F]	45
Potato pancakes—2 [Cal. %: 37 C, 4 P, 59 F]	220
Applesauce, unsweetened—½ cup [Cal. %: 98 C, 1 P, 1 F]	52
Total dinner calories	**572**

Evening Snack:

Navel orange [Cal. %: 92 C, 5 P, 3 F]	69
Dove dark chocolate–covered almonds—6 pieces [Cal. %: 43 C, 4 P, 53 F]	100
Total snack calories	**169**

Total daily calories—Day 6	**2,000**

DAY 7: 2000 Calorie Plan   Calorie Estimate

Note: Drink 8 oz. water with lemon/lime (0 Cal.) before all meals.

Breakfast:

Kashi flaxseed or blueberry waffles [Cal. %: 59 C, 11 P, 30 F]	150
Maple syrup—1 tbsp. [Cal. %: 99 C, 0 P, 1 F]	55
Egg—1 cooked with Pam [Cal. %: 2 C, 35 P, 63 F]	74
Orange juice—6 oz. [Cal. %: 95 C, 5 P, 0 F]	112
Total breakfast calories	**391**

Mid-Morning Snack:

Apple—1 medium [Cal. %: 90 C, 0 P, 10 F]	80
Hard cheese—1 oz. [Cal. %: 2 C, 29 P, 69 F]	130
Whole almonds—8 [Cal. %: 14 C, 14 P, 72 F]	56
Total snack calories	**266**

Lunch:

Turkey breast—5 oz. with lettuce [Cal. %: 0 C, 63 P, 37 F]	212
Cheddar cheese, 2%—1 slice [Cal. %: 4 C, 24 P, 72 F]	45
Rye bread—2 slices [Cal. %: 75 C, 14 P, 11 F]	130
Mustard—2 tspn. [Cal. %: 42 C, 21 P, 37 F]	6
Baby carrots—5 [Cal. %: 90 C, 7 P, 3 F]	16
Total lunch calories	**409**

Midday Snack:

Strawberries—1 cup [Cal. %: 86 C, 6 P, 8 F]	61
Walnuts, chopped—1/8 cup [Cal. %: 8 C, 8 P, 84 F]	100
Greek yogurt, 2%—6 oz. [Cal. %: 21 C, 52 P, 27 F]	120
Total snack calories	**281**

Dinner:

Flounder or sole—1 piece (6 oz.) [Cal. %: 1 C, 69 P, 30 F]	180
Baked potato, medium with 1 pat of butter [Cal. %: 60 C, 10 P, 30 F]	238
Green beans, cooked—1 cup [Cal. %: 77 C, 20 P, 3 F]	34
Extra virgin olive oil—1 tbsp. [Cal. %: 0 C, 0 P, 100 F]	100
Total dinner calories	**552**

Evening Snack:

Fat-free chocolate pudding cup [Cal. %: 84 C, 12 P, 4 F]	101
Total snack calories	**101**
Total daily calories—Day 7	**2,000**

Plan 2250: 2,250 Balanced-Calorie Seven-Day Eating Plan

DAY 1: 2250 Calorie Plan	Calorie Estimate

Note: Drink 8 oz. water with lemon/lime (0 Cal.) before all meals.

Breakfast:

Seven-grain waffles—2 [Cal. %: 62 C, 10 P, 28 F]	150
Maple syrup—2 tbsp. [Cal. %: 99 C, 0 P, 1 F]	104
Egg—1, cooked with Pam [Cal. %: 2 C, 35 P, 63 F]	74
Grapefruit juice—8 oz. [Cal. %: 95 C, 5 P, 0 F]	100
Total breakfast calories	**428**

Mid-Morning Snack:

Hard cheese—1 oz. [Cal. %: 2 C, 29 P, 69 F]	130
Whole almonds—1/4 cup [Cal. %: 14 C, 13 P, 73 F]	170
Total snack calories	**300**

Lunch:

Turkey breast—6 oz. [Cal. %: 0 C, 63 P, 37 F]	240
Rye bread—2 slices [Cal. %: 75 C, 14 P, 11 F]	130
Romaine lettuce—2 leaves [Cal. %: 75 C, 25 P, 0 F]	6
Light mayo—1 tbsp. [Cal. %: 15 C, 0 P, 85 F]	35
Baby carrots—3 [Cal. %: 90 C, 7 P, 3 F]	12
Total lunch calories	**423**

Midday Snack:

Peaches in light syrup—1 cup [Cal. %: 87 C, 8 P, 5 F]	210
Greek yogurt, 2%—6 oz. [Cal. %: 21 C, 52 P, 27 F]	120
Total snack calories	**330**

Dinner:

Flounder or sole—1 piece (6 oz.) [Cal. %: 1 C, 69 P, 30 F]	180
Baked potato—1 large with butter [Cal. %: 62 C, 8 P, 30 F]	245
Asparagus, fresh, steamed—8 spears [Cal. %: 36 C, 20 P, 44 F]	45
Grated Parmesan cheese—1 1/2 tbsp. [Cal. %: 0 C, 37 P, 63 F]	30
Extra virgin olive oil—1 tbsp. [Cal. %: 0 C, 0 P, 100 F]	100
Total dinner calories	**600**

Evening Snack:

Navel orange [Cal. %: 92 C, 5 P, 3 F]	69
Cottage cheese, 2%—4 oz. or 1/2 cup [Cal. %: 16 C, 65 P, 19 F]	100
Total snack calories	**169**

Total Daily Calories—Day 1	**2250**

DAY 2: 2250 Calorie Plan   Calorie Estimate

Note: Drink 8 oz. water with lemon/lime (0 Cal.) before all meals.

Breakfast:

Cheerios, plain—1¹/₂ cups [Cal. %: 70 C, 12 P, 18 F]	150
Skim milk—1 cup [Cal. %: 54 C, 41 P, 5 F]	86
Blueberries—1 cup [Cal. %: 92 C, 3 P, 5 F]	83
Orange juice—6 oz. [Cal. %: 95 C, 5 P, 0 F]	112
Total breakfast calories	**431**

Mid-Morning Snack:

Brown rice cakes—2 [Cal. %: 87 C, 7 P, 6 F]	70
Organic creamy peanut butter—1¹/₂ tbsp. [Cal. %: 12 C, 16 P, 72 F]	150
Skim milk—8 oz. [Cal. %: 51 C, 44 P, 5 F]	80
Total snack calories	**300**

Lunch:

Tuna fish—5 oz. [Cal. %: 0 C, 63 P, 37 F]	280
Romaine lettuce—4 leaves [Cal. %: 75 C, 25 P, 0 F]	12
Light Caesar dressing—2 tbsp. [Cal. %: 11 C, 5 P, 84 F]	80
Apple—1 medium [Cal. %: 90 C, 0 P, 10 F]	80
Total lunch calories	**452**

Midday Snack:

ZonePerfect Bar [Cal. %: 47 C, 21 P, 32 F]	200
Pear [Cal. %: 96 C, 2 P, 2 F]	96
Total snack calories	**296**

Dinner:

Chicken sausage—2 links [Cal. %: 6 C, 46 P, 48 F]	260
Whole-grain brown rice—1 cup [Cal. %: 84 C, 10 P, 6 F]	150
Steamed broccoli with lemon—³/₄ cup [Cal. %: 66 C, 25 P, 9 F]	30
Mixed green salad—1¹/₂ cups [Cal. %: 66 C, 26 P, 8 F]	16
Cranraisins—¹/₃ cup [Cal. %: 100 C, 0 P, 0 F]	130
Total dinner calories	**586**

Evening Snack:

Smartfood white cheddar popcorn [Cal. %: 37 C, 8 P, 55 F]	100
Mozzarella stick [Cal. %: 5 C, 35 P, 60 F]	85
Total snack calories	**185**

Total daily calories—Day 2	**2,250**

DAY 3: 2250 Calorie Plan	Calorie Estimate

Note: Drink 8 oz. water with lemon/lime (0 Cal.) before all meals.

Breakfast:

Steel-cut oatmeal—$1/2$ cup [Cal. %: 72 C, 13 P, 15 F]	300
Brown sugar—1 tspn. [Cal. %: 100 C, 0 P, 0 F]	15
Walnuts, chopped—$1/8$ cup [Cal. %: 8 C, 8 P, 84 F]	100
Peach—1 medium [Cal. %: 87 C, 8 P, 5 F]	38
Total breakfast calories	**453**

Mid-Morning Snack:

Cottage cheese, 2%—6 oz. [Cal. %: 16 C, 65 P, 19 F]	150
Walnuts, chopped—$1/8$ cup [Cal. %: 8 C, 8 P, 84 F]	100
Pineapple—2 slices, $3/4$-inch thick [Cal. %: 95 C, 3 P, 2 F]	80
Total snack calories	**330**

Lunch:

Turkey burger, lettuce, and tomato—6 oz. [Cal. %: 10 C, 35 P, 55 F]	390
Whole-wheat pita—1 medium [Cal. %: 80 C, 15 P, 5 F]	123
Ketchup—1 tbsp. [Cal. %: 100 C, 0 P, 0 F]	20
Baby carrots—6 [Cal. %: 90 C, 7 P, 3 F]	24
Total lunch calories	**557**

Midday Snack:

Pear [Cal. %: 96 C, 2 P, 2 F]	96
Kashi Bar [Cal. %: 43 C, 4 P, 53 F]	130
Total snack calories	**226**

Dinner:

Whole-wheat spaghetti—$1^1/2$ cups [Cal. %: 81 C, 15 P, 4 F]	278
Chicken (or vegetable) broth—$1^1/2$ cups [Cal. %: 50 C, 28 P, 22 F]	18
Chickpeas—$1/2$ cup [Cal. %: 67 C, 20 P, 13 F]	100
Shrimp—8 [Cal. %: 0 C, 100 P, 0 F]	94
Fresh parsley, chopped—1 cup [Cal. %: 63 C, 19 P, 18 F]	22
Total dinner calories	**512**

Evening Snack:

Vanilla soy milk [Cal. %: 52 C, 23 P, 25 F]	110
Raspberries—1 cup [Cal. %: 83 C, 7 P, 10 F]	62
Total snack calories	**172**

Total daily calories—Day 3	**2,250**

DAY 4: 2250 Calorie Plan   Calorie Estimate

Note: Drink 8 oz. water with lemon/lime (0 Cal.) before all meals.

Breakfast:

Oat-bran English muffin—1 [Cal. %: 72 C, 15 P, 13 F]	150
Eggs—2 large, scrambled, cooked with Pam [Cal. %: 5 C, 29 P, 66 F]	154
Grapefruit—half [Cal. %: 91 C, 6 P, 3 F]	52
Total breakfast calories	**356**

Mid-Morning Snack:

Hummus—2¹/₂ tbsp. [Cal. %: 45 C, 11 P, 44 F]	67
Carrots, celery, tomatoes, peppers—1¹/₂ cups [Cal. %: 82 C, 10 P, 8 F]	100
Reduced-fat ranch dressing—2 tbsp. [Cal. %: 28 C, 2 P, 70 F]	70
Total snack calories	**237**

Lunch:

Grilled chicken breast—6 oz. [Cal. %: 0 C, 63 P, 37 F]	330
Low-fat cheddar cheese—1 slice [Cal. %: 0 C, 44 P, 56 F]	70
Romaine lettuce—4 leaves [Cal. %: 75 C, 25 P, 0 F]	12
Organic blue corn chips—6 chips [Cal. %: 55 C, 6 P, 39 F]	140
Baby carrots—6 [Cal. %: 90 C, 7 P, 3 F]	24
Total lunch calories	**576**

Midday Snack:

Apple—1 medium [Cal. %: 90 C, 0 P, 10 F]	80
Organic peanut butter—2 tbsp. [Cal. %: 12 C, 16 P, 72 F]	200
Total snack calories	**280**

Dinner:

Split-pea soup—2 cups [Cal. %: 64 C, 20 P, 16 F]	330
Croutons—³/₄ cup [Cal. %: 55 C, 9 P, 36 F]	140
Mozzarella cheese, part skim—2 sticks [Cal. %: 5 C, 35 P, 60 F]	170
Total dinner calories	**640**

Evening Snack:

Applesauce, unsweetened—1¹/₂ cups [Cal. %: 98 C, 1 P, 1 F]	156
Cinnamon, 1 tspn. [Cal. %: 87 C, 3 P, 10 F]	5
Total snack calories	**161**

Total daily calories—Day 4	**2,250**

DAY 5: 2250 Calorie Plan   Calorie Estimate

Note: Drink 8 oz. water with lemon/lime (0 Cal.) before all meals.

Breakfast:

French toast—2 slices [Cal. %: 60 C, 15 P, 25 F]	252
Maple syrup—2 tbsp. [Cal. %: 99 C, 0 P, 1 F]	104
V8 Vegetable Juice—1 cup [Cal. %: 75 C, 18 P, 7 F]	72
Total breakfast calories	**428**

Mid-Morning Snack:

Greek yogurt, 2%, with fruit—1 cup or 8 oz. [Cal. %: 22 C, 54 P, 24 F]	140
Banana—1 medium [Cal. %: 92 C, 5 P, 3 F]	105
Total snack calories	**245**

Lunch:

Egg-white salad with light mayo and chives—1/2 cup [Cal. %: 15 C, 52 P, 33 F]	260
Rye bread—2 slices [Cal. %: 75 C, 14 P, 11 F]	130
Romaine lettuce—2 leaves [Cal. %: 75 C, 25 P, 0 F]	6
Cantaloupe—1 cup [Cal. %: 86 C, 9 P, 5 F]	60
Blueberries—1/2 cup [Cal. %: 92 C, 3 P, 5 F]	42
Total lunch calories	**498**

Midday Snack:

Whole almonds—1/4 cup [Cal. %: 14 C, 13 P, 73 F]	170
Dried figs—3 [Cal. %: 14 C, 13 P, 73 F]	141
Total snack calories	**311**

Dinner:

Lasagna with meat—1 piece (3 x 4 in.) [Cal. %: 42 C, 25 P, 33 F]	336
Italian bread–2 medium pieces [Cal. %: 76 C, 13 P, 11 F]	108
Mixed green salad—1½ cups [Cal. %: 55 C, 9 P, 36 F]	15
Olive oil dressing—1 tbsp. and lemon juice—1 tbsp. [Cal. %: 2 C, 0 P, 98 F]	111
Total dinner calories	**570**

Evening Snack:

Navel orange [Cal. %: 92 C, 5 P, 3 F]	69
Skim milk—1 cup [Cal. %: 54 C, 41 P, 5 F]	129
Total snack calories	**198**

Total daily calories—Day 5	**2,250**

DAY 6: 2250 Calorie Plan	Calorie Estimate

Note: Drink 8 oz. water with lemon/lime (0 Cal.) before all meals.

Breakfast:

Soy protein shake—1½ scoops [Cal. %: 51 C, 42 P, 7 F]	195
Plain yogurt, 1%—1 cup [Cal. %: 45 C, 33 P, 22 F]	140
Mixed berries, frozen or fresh—1½ cups [Cal. %: 94 C, 6 P, 0 F]	105
Total breakfast calories	**440**

Mid-Morning Snack:

Rye bread—1 slice [Cal. %: 75 C, 14 P, 11 F]	65
Organic peanut butter—2 tbsp. [Cal. %: 12 C, 16 P, 72 F]	200
Reduced-sugar raspberry jelly—1 tbsp. [Cal. %: 100 C, 0 P, 0 F]	35
Total snack calories	**300**

Lunch:

Turkey breast—6 oz. [Cal. %: 15 C, 52 P, 33 F]	240
Cheddar cheese, 2%—2 slices [Cal. %: 0 C, 44 P, 56 F]	140
Romaine lettuce—3 leaves [Cal. %: 75 C, 25 P, 0 F]	9
Apple—1 medium [Cal. %: 90 C, 0 P, 10 F]	80
Total lunch calories	**469**

Midday Snack:

Pear—1 medium [Cal. %: 96 C, 2 P, 2 F]	96
Cheese stick, light [Cal. %: 0 C, 44 P, 56 F]	45
Pistachios—½ cup with shells [Cal. %: 10 C, 15 P, 75 F]	160
Total snack calories	**301**

Dinner:

Rotisserie chicken—6 oz. [Cal. %: 0 C, 47 P, 53 F]	225
Sweet potato—1 medium [Cal. %: 94 C, 6 P, 0 F]	112
Butter (for sweet potato)—1 tbsp. [Cal. %: 0 C, 1 P, 99 F]	102
Mixed green salad—1½ cup [Cal. %: 66 C, 26 P, 8 F]	15
Olive oil dressing—1 tbsp. with lemon juice—1 tbsp. [Cal. %: 2 C, 0 P, 98 F]	111
Total dinner calories	**565**

Evening Snack:

Dove dark chocolate–covered almonds—6 pieces [Cal. %: 43 C, 4 P, 53 F]	100
Cherries, fresh—1 cup [Cal. %: 91 C, 6 P, 3 F]	75
Total snack calories	**175**

Total daily calories—Day 6	**2,250**

DAY 7: 2250 Calorie Plan — Calorie Estimate

Note: Drink 8 oz. water with lemon/lime (0 Cal.) before all meals.

Breakfast:

Omelet—2 medium eggs, cooked with Pam [Cal. %: 2 C, 35 P, 63 F]	150
Chopped potato, medium, browned in Pam [Cal. %: 91 C, 8 P, 1 F]	142
Cheddar cheese, 2%—1 slice [Cal. %: 0 C, 44 P, 56 F]	70
Orange juice—6 oz. [Cal. %: 95 C, 5 P, 0 F]	112
Total breakfast calories	**474**

Mid-Morning Snack:

Whole almonds—20 [Cal. %: 14 C, 13 P, 73 F]	140
Raisins—1/4 cup [Cal. %: 95 C, 4 P, 1 F]	109
Total snack calories	**249**

Lunch:

California sushi roll—4 pieces [Cal. %: 67 C, 11 P, 22 F]	300
Miso soup—2 cups [Cal. %: 36 C, 29 P, 35 F]	168
Navel orange [Cal. %: 92 C, 5 P, 3 F]	69
Total lunch calories	**537**

Midday Snack:

Apple—1 medium [Cal. %: 90 C, 0 P, 10 F]	80
Organic peanut butter—2 tbsp. [Cal. %: 12 C, 16 P, 72 F]	200
Total snack calories	**280**

Dinner:

Whole-wheat pasta—1 1/2 cups [Cal. %: 80 C, 16 P, 4 F]	255
Sun-dried tomatoes—3 pieces [Cal. %: 43 C, 9 P, 48 F]	45
Broccoli, cooked—1 cup [Cal. %: 70 C, 21 P, 9 F]	35
Black olives, medium, pitted—7 [Cal. %: 15 C, 0 P, 85 F]	35
Extra virgin olive oil—1 tbsp. [Cal. %: 0 C, 0 P, 100 F]	100
Italian bread—1 medium piece [Cal. %: 76 C, 13 P, 11 F]	54
Total dinner calories	**524**

Evening Snack:

Graham cracker—1 [Cal. %: 73 C, 6 P, 21 F]	30
Low-fat vanilla yogurt—3/4 cup [Cal. %: 73 C, 6 P, 21 F]	156
Total snack calories	**186**

Total daily calories—Day 7	**2,250**

Plan 2500: 2,500 Balanced-Calorie Seven-Day Eating Plan

DAY 1: 2500 Calorie Plan	Calorie Estimate

Note: Drink 8 oz. water with lemon/lime (0 Cal.) before all meals.

Breakfast:

Greek yogurt, 2%, plain—1¹/₂ cups [Cal. %: 22 C, 54 P, 24 F]	210
Almonds, sliced—¹/₄ cup [Cal. %: 14 C, 13 P, 73 F]	134
Blueberries—³/₄ cup [Cal. %: 92 C, 3 P, 5 F]	63
Grapefruit juice—8 oz. [Cal. %: 95 C, 5 P, 0 F]	100
Total breakfast calories	**507**

Mid-Morning Snack:

Apple—1 medium [Cal. %: 90 C, 0 P, 10 F]	80
Cheese stick, light—3 [Cal. %: 0 C, 44 P, 56 F]	135
Smartfood white cheddar popcorn [Cal. %: 37 C, 8 P, 55 F]	100
Total snack calories	**315**

Lunch:

Field greens or spinach—2 cups [Cal. %: 61 C, 29 P, 10 F]	68
Grilled chicken breast—6 oz. [Cal. %: 0 C, 63 P, 37 F]	330
Feta cheese—¹/₄ cup [Cal. %: 7 C, 40 P, 53 F]	75
Pear [Cal. %: 96 C, 2 P, 2 F]	96
Total lunch calories	**569**

Midday Snack:

Organic peanut butter—2 tbsp. [Cal. %: 12 C, 16 P, 72 F]	200
Wasa Light Rye Crispbread—2 crackers [Cal. %: 91 C, 9 P, 0 F]	60
Celery (4 sticks) and baby carrots (5) [Cal. %: 76 C, 14 P, 10 F]	40
Total snack calories	**300**

Dinner:

Lentil soup—2 cups [Cal. %: 56 C, 19 P, 25 F]	360
Firm tofu—6 oz. [Cal. %: 15 C, 46 P, 39 F]	150
Frozen stir-fry vegetables—1¹/₂ cups [Cal. %: 83 C, 17 P, 0 F]	59
Extra virgin olive oil—1 tbsp.[Cal. %: 0 C, 0 P, 100 F]	100
Total dinner calories	**669**

Evening Snack:

Weight Watchers ice cream—6 oz. [Cal. %: 43 C, 4 P, 53 F]	140
Total snack calories	**140**

Total daily calories—Day 1	**2500**

DAY 2: 2500 Calorie Plan   Calorie Estimate

Note: Drink 8 oz. water with lemon/lime (0 Cal.) before all meals.

Breakfast:

Oat-bran English muffin—1 [Cal. %: 72 C, 15 P, 13 F]	125
Almond butter—1/2 tbsp. [Cal. %: 13 C, 8 P, 79 F]	100
Cottage cheese, 2%—1 cup [Cal. %: 16 C, 65 P, 19 F]	200
Cantaloupe—1 cup [Cal. %: 86 C, 9 P, 5F]	60
Total breakfast calories	**485**

Mid-Morning Snack:

Whole almonds—20 [Cal. %: 14 C, 13 P, 73 F]	140
Raisins—1/4 cup [Cal. %: 95 C, 4 P, 1 F]	109
Dried mango—4 strips [Cal. %: 96 C, 2 P, 2 F]	55
Total snack calories	**304**

Lunch:

Lean beef or turkey burger—6 oz. [Cal. %: 4 C, 69 P, 27 F]	240
Rye bread—2 slices [Cal. %: 75 C, 14 P, 11 F]	130
Ketchup—2 tbsp. [Cal. %: 100 C, 0 P, 0 F]	40
Field greens [Cal. %: 80 C, 20 P, 0 F]	30
Baked lentil chips—11 chips [Cal. %: 64 C, 13 P, 23 F]	55
Apple juice—1 cup [Cal. %: 100 C, 0 P, 0 F]	117
Total lunch calories	**612**

Midday Snack:

Hard-boiled eggs—2 [Cal. %: 3 C, 33 P, 64 F]	154
Navel orange (1) and grapes (1/2 cup) [Cal. %: 92 C, 5 P, 3 F]	152
Total snack calories	**306**

Dinner:

Chicken sausage—2 links or 6 oz. [Cal. %: 4 C, 42 P, 54 F]	280
Whole-wheat pasta—1 cup [Cal. %: 80 C, 16 P, 4 F]	170
Broccoli with diced tomatoes—1 1/2 cups, cooked [Cal. %: 70 C, 21 P, 9 F]	107
Extra virgin olive oil—1 tbsp. [Cal. %: 0 C, 0 P, 100 F]	100
Total dinner calories	**657**

Evening Snack:

Skim milk—1 cup [Cal. %: 54 C, 41 P, 5 F]	86
Swiss Miss fat-free hot chocolate [Cal. %: 76 C, 24 P, 0 F]	50
Total snack calories	**136**

Total daily calories—Day 2	**2,500**

DAY 3: 2500 Calorie Plan   Calorie Estimate

Note: Drink 8 oz. water with lemon/lime (0 Cal.) before all meals.

Breakfast:

Kashi blueberry flaxseed waffles—3 [Cal. %: 59 C, 11 P, 30 F]	225
Maple syrup—2 tbsp. [Cal. %: 99 C, 0 P, 1 F]	104
Eggs—2, cooked with Pam [Cal. %: 2 C, 35 P, 63 F]	154
Coffee with cream [Cal. %: 13 C, 9 P, 78 F]	26
Total breakfast calories	**509**

Mid-Morning Snack:

Vegetable juice (V8 low-sodium) 8 oz. [Cal. %: 83 C, 17 P, 0 F]	50
Wasa Multi-Grain Cracker—2 [Cal. %: 91 C, 9 P. 0 F]	90
Hummus—4 tbsp. [Cal. %: 45 C, 11 P, 44 F]	162
Total snack calories	**302**

Lunch:

Bumble Bee Tuna Medley, Lemon Pepper—6 oz. [Cal. %: 7 C, 68 P, 25 F]	220
Multigrain brown rice cakes—4 [Cal. %: 85 C, 7 P, 8 F]	140
Baby spinach—2 cups with honey mustard [Cal. %: 35 C, 20 P, 45 F]	89
Apple—1 medium [Cal. %: 90 C, 0 P, 10 F]	80
Baby carrots—6 [Cal. %: 90 C, 7 P, 3 F]	24
Total lunch calories	**553**

Midday Snack:

Clif Mojo Bar [Cal. %: 32 C, 18P, 50 F]	200
Greek yogurt, 2%—5 oz. [Cal. %: 21 C, 52 P, 27 F]	100
Total snack calories	**300**

Dinner:

Lean turkey chili with beans—1¹/₂ cups [Cal. %: 36 C, 34 P, 34 F]	330
Cheddar cheese, 2%, on top—2 slices [Cal. %: 4 C, 24 P, 72 F]	90
Tostitos blue corn chips—6 big chips [Cal. %: 55 C, 6 P, 39 F]	140
Mixed green salad—1¹/₂ cups [Cal. %: 66 C, 26 P, 8 F]	15
Olive oil dressing—¹/₂ tbsp. with lemon [Cal. %: 2 C, 0 P, 98 F]	50
Total dinner calories	**625**

Evening Snack:

Applesauce, unsweetened—1 cup [Cal. %: 98 C, 1 P, 1 F]	104
Cinnamon—1 tspn. [Cal. %: 87 C, 3 P, 10 F]	6
Hard cheese—1 oz. [Cal. %: 4 C, 28 P, 68 F]	101
Total snack calories	**211**

Total daily calories—Day 3	**2,500**

DAY 4: 2500 Calorie Plan	Calorie Estimate

Note: Drink 8 oz. water with lemon/lime (0 Cal.) before all meals.

Breakfast:

Steel-cut oatmeal—¹/₂ cup [Cal. %: 72 C, 13 P, 15 F]	300
Blueberries—¹/₂ cup [Cal. %: 92 C, 3 P, 5 F]	42
Walnuts, chopped—¹/₈ cup [Cal. %: 8 C, 8 P, 84 F]	100
Orange juice—6 oz. [Cal. %: 95 C, 5 P, 0 F]	112
Total breakfast calories	**554**

Mid-Morning Snack:

Laughing Cow Swiss cheese—3 wedges [Cal. %: 16 C, 31 P, 53 F]	105
Whole-wheat pita—1 medium [Cal. %: 80 C, 15 P, 5 F]	123
Apple—1 medium [Cal. %: 90 C, 0 P, 10 F]	80
Total snack calories	**308**

Lunch:

Boca Burger, flame-grilled [Cal. %: 19 C, 45 P, 36 F]	120
Corn tortilla (6-inch)—2 [Cal. %: 82 C, 7 P, 11 F]	120
Mixed greens, sliced tomatoes—1¹/₂ cups [Cal. %: 66 C, 26 P, 8 F]	25
Olive oil / balsamic vinegar dressing—1 tbsp. [Cal. %: 2 C, 0 P, 98 F]	116
Cranraisins—¹/₂ oz. [Cal. %: 100 C, 0 P, 0 F]	50
Sunflower seeds, shelled—¹/₈ cup [Cal. %: 11 C, 19 P, 71 F]	95
Total lunch calories	**526**

Midday Snack:

Dove dark chocolate–covered almonds—4 pieces [Cal. %: 43 C, 4 P, 53 F]	67
Applesauce, unsweetened—1¹/₂ cups [Cal. %: 98 C, 1 P, 1 F]	172
Total snack calories	**239**

Dinner:

Potato-crusted fish fillets—3 (3.4 oz.) [Cal. %: 18 C, 22 P, 60 F]	405
Whole-grain brown rice—1 cup [Cal. %: 84 C, 10 P, 6 F]	215
Steamed broccoli with fresh-squeezed lemon [Cal. %: 66 C, 25 P, 9 F]	41
Total dinner calories	**661**

Evening Snack:

Vanilla soy milk—1¹/₂ cups [Cal. %: 52 C, 23 P, 25 F]	150
Raspberries—1 cup [Cal. %: 83 C, 7 P, 10 F]	62
Total snack calories	**212**
Total daily calories—Day 4	**2,500**

DAY 5: 2500 Calorie Plan — Calorie Estimate

Note: Drink 8 oz. water with lemon/lime (0 Cal.) before all meals.

Breakfast:

Oat-bran hot cereal—³/₄ cup [Cal. %: 65 C, 18 P, 17 F]	225
Peaches in light syrup—1 cup [Cal. %: 87 C, 8 P, 5 F]	138
Latte coffee [Cal. %: 39 C, 27 P, 34 F]	142
Total breakfast calories	**505**

Mid-Morning Snack:

Goat cheese, hard—1.5 oz. [Cal. %: 2 C, 29 P, 69 F]	192
Grapes, seedless—1 cup [Cal. %: 94 C, 4 P, 2 F]	110
Total snack calories	**302**

Lunch:

Egg-white salad with light mayo and chives—¹/₂ cup [Cal. %: 15 C, 52 P, 33 F]	260
Mission large flour tortilla—1 [Cal. %: 69 C, 11 P, 20 F]	210
Pear [Cal. %: 96 C, 2 P, 2 F]	96
Total lunch calories	**566**

Midday Snack:

Banana—1 medium [Cal. %: 92 C, 5 P, 3 F]	105
Whole almonds—20 [Cal. %: 14 C, 14 P, 72 F]	140
Raisins—¹/₄ cup [Cal. %: 95 C, 4 P, 1 F]	109
Total snack calories	**354**

Dinner:

Split-pea soup—2 cups [Cal. %: 72 C, 28 P, 0 F]	200
Wasa Whole-Grain Crispbread—4 crackers [Cal. %: 91 C, 9 P, 0 F]	160
Grated Parmesan cheese—1.5 oz. [Cal. %: 4 C, 38 P, 58 F]	183
Total dinner calories	**543**

Evening Snack:

Pineapple—2 slices, ³/₄-inch-thick [Cal. %: 95 C, 3 P, 2 F]	80
Cottage cheese, 2%—³/₄ cup [Cal. %: 16 C, 65 P, 19 F]	150
Total snack calories	**230**

Total daily calories—Day 5	**2,500**

DAY 6: 2500 Calorie Plan	Calorie Estimate

Note: Drink 8 oz. water with lemon/lime (0 Cal.) before all meals.

Breakfast:

Whole-grain bread, toasted—2 slices [Cal. %: 69 C, 19 P, 12 F]	220
Reduced-sugar raspberry jelly—2 tbsp. [Cal. %: 100 C, 0 P, 0 F]	70
Light cream cheese—3 tbsp. [Cal. %: 15 C, 16 P, 69 F]	90
Grapefruit juice—8 oz. [Cal. %: 95 C, 5 P, 0 F]	100
Coffee with cream [Cal. %: 13 C, 9 P, 78 F]	50
Total breakfast calories	**530**

Mid-Morning Snack:

Fruit and nut trail mix—4 tbsp. [Cal. %: 36 C, 8 P, 56 F]	186
Greek yogurt, 2%—6 oz. [Cal. %: 21 C, 52 P, 27 F]	120
Total snack calories	**306**

Lunch:

Tuna fish (6 oz.) with 2 leaves of lettuce [Cal. %: 18 C, 80 P, 2 F]	150
Light mayo—2 tbsp. [Cal. %: 15 C, 0 P, 85 F]	70
Multigrain brown rice cakes—4 [Cal. %: 85 C, 7 P, 8 F]	140
Baby carrots—6 [Cal. %: 90 C, 7 P, 3 F]	24
Apple—1 medium [Cal. %: 90 C, 0 P, 10 F]	80
Total lunch calories	**464**

Midday Snack:

Pear [Cal. %: 96 C, 2 P, 2 F]	96
Whole-wheat pita—1 medium [Cal. %: 80 C, 15 P, 5 F]	123
Laughing Cow Swiss cheese—3 wedges [Cal. %: 16 C, 31 P, 53 F]	105
Total snack calories	**324**

Dinner:

Roasted white-meat chicken—6 oz. [Cal. %: 0 C, 38 P, 62 F]	320
Sweet potato with 1 pat of butter [Cal. %: 50 C, 4 P, 46 F]	214
Boston lettuce (1 cup) with lite dressing (1 tbsp.) [Cal. %: 55 C, 33 P, 12 F]	65
Brussels sprouts with lemon—1 1/2 cups [Cal. %: 74 C, 20 P, 6 F]	57
Total dinner calories	**656**

Evening Snack:

Fat-free chocolate-vanilla swirl pudding snack [Cal. %: 92 C, 8 P, 0 F]	100
Ginger snaps—3 cookies [Cal. %: 74 C, 3 P, 23 F]	120
Total snack calories	**220**

Total daily calories—Day 6	**2,500**

DAY 7: 2500 Calorie Plan — Calorie Estimate

Note: Drink 8 oz. water with lemon/lime (0 Cal.) before all meals.

Breakfast:
Spinach omelet—2 medium eggs, cooked with Pam [Cal. %: 2 C, 35 P, 63 F]	200
Multigrain English muffin with jelly [Cal. %: 71 C, 13 P, 16 F]	220
Coffee with cream [Cal. %: 13 C, 9 P, 78 F]	50
Total breakfast calories	**470**

Mid-Morning Snack:
Banana (1 large) and strawberries (1 cup) [Cal. %: 92 C, 5 P, 3 F]	156
Light Muscle Milk, chocolate [Cal. %: 16 C, 61 P, 23 F]	100
Total snack calories	**256**

Lunch:
Chicken salad with light mayo—6 oz. [Cal. %: 0 C, 63 P, 37 F]	370
Simply Naked pita chips—1 oz. (or about 10 chips)[Cal. %: 55 C, 10 P, 35 F]	130
Apple—1 medium [Cal. %: 90 C, 0 P, 10 F]	80
Total lunch calories	**580**

Midday Snack:
Cottage cheese, 2%—1/2 cup [Cal. %: 16 C, 65 P, 19 F]	150
Pineapple—2 slices, 3/4-inch thick [Cal. %: 95 C, 3 P, 2 F]	80
Whole almonds—10 [Cal. %: 14 C, 13 P, 73 F]	70
Total snack calories	**300**

Dinner:
Grilled flounder or sole—6 oz. [Cal. %: 1 C, 69 P, 30 F]	226
Baked potato—1 large, with 1 pat of butter [Cal. %: 62 C, 8 P, 30 F]	245
Mixed greens and asparagus—1 1/2 cups [Cal. %: 66 C, 26 P, 8 F]	55
Green beans, cooked—1 cup [Cal. %: 77 C, 20 P, 3 F]	37
Extra virgin olive oil—1 tbsp. [Cal. %: 0 C, 0 P, 100 F]	100
Total dinner calories	**663**

Evening Snack:
Vanilla soy milk—8 oz. [Cal. %: 52 C, 23 P, 25 F]	120
Raspberries—1 cup [Cal. %: 83 C, 7 P, 10 F]	62
Dove dark chocolate-covered almonds—3 pieces [Cal. %: 43 C, 4 P, 53 F]	49
Total snack calories	**231**
Total daily calories—Day 7	**2,500**

CHAPTER 6

Winning Hydration for Endurance Athletes

> To win without risk is to
> triumph without glory.
>
> —*Pierre Corneille*

The Importance of Hydration for Endurance Athletes

While it is now common knowledge that proper hydration is key for optimal endurance sports performance, it is still surprising how the vast majority of athletes get this wrong.

Some athletes pay very little attention to hydration during training. When they get to the race, not only do they lack a good hydration plan, but they also have little understanding of their own unique hydration needs. There are athletes who do practice hydration in training and develop a race plan, but then on the big day, in the excitement of competition, they fail to follow it. Still others have a plan worked out, but then at the last minute hear some marketing hype about a new plan a famous athlete is using and they decide to try it out. This is a classic "rookie mistake." Race day is not a day for experimentation.

Hydration is so important that from a coaching standpoint, it's the first thing we ask about if an athlete's race performance falls short of expectations. Fueling is second, but we will cover that in the next chapter. When an athlete is confused about what went wrong in a race, we first ask them exactly what, how much, and when they drank, before and during the race. It is amazing how often this question quickly gets us on the right track to finding the problem and then determining what we need to do to fix it.

Oftentimes, an athlete believes he or she has sufficiently hydrated before and during the competition, but when we then analyze what actually happened, we find that it is not so. For this reason, it is very important to determine your hydration needs in advance, test and practice your proper hydration routine during training, and then stick to it on race day. And the longer the race, the more critical hydration becomes. As we like to joke about with ultras and other longer races, hydration and fueling errors are measured in hours, not minutes.

Hydrating by "Feel"

We do receive pushback from time to time on the importance of planning hydration with such accuracy and detail. Many believe that your body will "tell" you when it's thirsty, and all you really need to do is listen to it. There is some truth to this theory, and in fact, we often find that most athletes don't listen to their bodies enough. Yet when it comes to hydration, "feel" alone does not work. There is just too much of a delay in the time between when your hydration is actually running low and when you first feel thirsty. In fact, when it comes to competition, the delay is so long that by the time you start to feel thirsty, you are probably already dangerously low on hydration, and it will be difficult, if not impossible, to bring your hydration levels back to where they need to be.

Unfortunately, hydrating by feel doesn't work in endurance sports. We need to know our proper hydration levels, develop a hydration plan to satisfy them, practice our plan in training, and then execute our plan on race day.

Cardiovascular Drift

There is an optimal level of hydration for each athlete that allows him or her to perform at their best. As hydration levels decrease from this amount, an athlete's performance either decreases at the same level of effort, or the athlete has to work much harder to maintain the same level of performance, thus elevating his heart rate. This effect is known as *cardiovascular drift.*

For example, if a well-trained athlete runs at an even pace for an hour at a constant aerobic heart rate (75% of maximum) in a relatively cool temperature (60°F), and he hydrates well before and throughout his run, his heart rate is likely to stay right around that same level for the entire hour.

If, on the other hand, the same well-trained athlete does the same experiment but fails to hydrate well before and throughout his run, his heart rate will likely either need to increase to maintain the same pace as the run progresses, or his pace will have to slow to maintain the same heart rate.

External heat is a significant factor in your performance because it affects your body's ability to cool itself down. So, in the same example, all other factors being the same, if we increase the temperature to 90 degrees Fahrenheit, proper hydration becomes even more critical as the potential impact of cardiovascular drift increases substantially. The athlete who did not hydrate well before and throughout would see an even greater effect. His or her heart rate would have to push even higher to maintain the same pace, or he or she would have to go much slower to maintain the same heart rate.

The really interesting point to note is that the hydrated athlete would probably also experience some level of cardiovascular drift, too, unless he or she increased hydration levels to compensate for the increase in heat. This is because the amount of fluid to keep properly hydrated at 60 degrees Fahrenheit would probably be insufficient at 90 degrees Fahrenheit.

Determining Your Own Unique Hydration Needs

The easiest way to determine your body's own unique hydration needs is through proper testing in training. We have developed a simple "Sweat Rate Test" that we have successfully used over the years with athletes we coach.

Our Sweat Rate Test protocol is as follows:

Sweat Rate Test

1. Weigh yourself (without clothing) just prior to beginning your endurance activity (e.g., run, cycle, swim, etc.).
2. Do your endurance activity for 60 minutes at a heart rate equal to 75 percent of your maximum heart rate (MHR).
3. During the 60 minutes of activity, very evenly consume 16 ounces of water.
4. Weigh yourself (without clothing) immediately after your 60-minute activity has been completed.
5. Complete the following calculations:

   - Weight Before – Weight After = Net Weight Loss
   - Net Weight Loss + 1.0 pound (16 oz. of water consumed) = Hourly Sweat Loss
     Note: 1 pound = 16 ounces

Athlete Example: Sweat Rate Test

The following example applies the Sweat Rate Test protocol to an athlete who weighs 165.0 pounds before the test and 164.0 pounds after the test. Following is the calculation:

Weight Before = 165.0 pounds

Weight After = 164.0 pounds

1. Weight Loss: 165.0 – 164.0 = 1.0 pound (16 oz.)
2. Hourly Sweat Rate: 1.0 pound (16 oz.) + 1.0 pound (16 oz. of water consumed) = 2.0 pounds (32 oz.)

The athlete lost 16 ounces, despite replenishing with 16 ounces of fluid. Therefore, he is down a total of 32 ounces for the hour. This indicates that under similar conditions (i.e., temperature, heart rate level, and activity), he or she should replenish fluids at a rate of about 32 ounces per hour.

This is a great starting point, and it begins to give the athlete an idea of what his or her hydration needs are, and how to plan hydration replacement for training sessions and races.

But what if the conditions on race day are different? What if it's hotter?

For example, say the above test was conducted in fairly moderate temperatures of 60 degrees Fahrenheit. It would be wise to repeat the test in hotter conditions to get a better idea of how the athlete's needs change. Perhaps when the test is repeated at 90 degrees, the athlete gets a result of 48 ounces (3.0 pounds) per hour. This would suggest that in temperatures ranging from 60 degrees to 90 degrees, this athlete's hydration needs range from 32 ounces to 48 ounces per hour. This is extremely valuable information to have on race-day morning when you want to adjust your exact hydration strategy for the race.

Our suggestion to our coached athletes is to conduct this test several times over the year, and in varying conditions. By doing so, an athlete can plot a rough chart of his or her hydration needs that will serve as a guide when planning hydration for any race or training session.

Following is an example of what that might look like:

Temperature Fluid Replacement

(Degrees Fahrenheit)	(Ounces per Hour)
60 degrees	32 oz.
70 degrees	37 oz.
80 degrees	43 oz.
90 degrees	48 oz.

We also encourage athletes to test their sweat rates at different heart rates, including anticipated race pace heart rates. The above tests were done at 75 percent of MHR. There may be slight differences in sweat rate at higher or lower heart rates.

Likewise, we encourage athletes to test for other sports, too. For example, a triathlete may find that his running sweat rate differs from his cycling sweat rate.

In general, however, our suggestion to athletes is not to do a Sweat Rate Test only once or twice and think you have it nailed. Make it part of your regular training, and include it in many different training scenarios. The information you glean from this test will be very helpful when planning out your optimal race-day hydration, no matter what the conditions and situation.

Hyponatremia

While it is far more common to underhydrate than to overhydrate, overhydration is a risk that all endurance athletes should be aware of. Overhydration can result in a serious medical condition known as hyponatremia, an electrolyte disturbance in which sodium levels dilute well below normal.

While fairly rare, this potential health risk is another good reason to know your body's hydration needs in all situations, and to plan your training and racing hydration routines accordingly.

In the next chapter, we will explore why energy drinks—with carbohydrates, sodium, and other electrolytes—are often superior to water alone. Energy drinks, especially those with higher sodium content, will not dilute your body's sodium and other electrolyte levels as straight water can.

Hydration Logistics: What, When, Where, and How?

The topic of hydration logistics is often barely considered and even over-looked by many athletes. Once we decide on what plan we're going to use to hydrate, how much we plan to consume, and when we plan to consume it, it's not as if everything then just magically appears when you need it on race day. We need to have a well-thought-out logistical plan to go along with our hydration plan, and we need to practice it as part of our training regimen so that we can execute it flawlessly on race day.

The biggest problem area is often with fluids. A typical rookie mistake is that an athlete will often choose a particular energy drink to use in practice, but then in the week before the race, he or she realizes that the marathon course serves a different energy drink.

As we will discuss further in the next chapter, the important point to keep in mind for now is that an energy drink, since it has calories in it, is both a hydration source and a fueling source, which needs to be accounted for as you construct your fueling and hydration plan.

Citing the example above, what are your options if you have been training with a particular energy drink but you find that it will not be available at the race?

Probably the most common response to this question for most athletes is just to ignore it. In other words, just show up on race day and use the energy drink that the race provides and hope for the best. Some of the time you may get lucky and this will work out fine; but what if the drink doesn't appeal to you, so you have difficulty consuming enough of it—or, worse yet, what if it doesn't agree with you and makes you feel ill during the race? This will ruin your race and make the last three months of marathon preparation seem like a complete waste.

Again, race day is not a time for experimentation. Everything you do in a race should be tested and retested during training before relying on it on race day. We're talking about everything from equipment to race clothing to pre-race routines. However, in no area is testing and retesting more impor-tant than when it comes to what we put in our bodies before and during our races.

What we suggest to our coached athletes is that they should check the race website at least a couple of months in advance to find out what hydration sources will be available on the course, and also how frequently they will be available (i.e., determine how far apart the aid stations will be spaced from one another). We can then use this valuable information in our training. I encourage my athletes to get a supply of the stated race-day energy drink and to start practicing with it in training.

For the marathon, the best time to practice race-day hydration is during the weekly long run. We will typically have our coached athletes consume the race energy drink during their long runs, and to do so in the same quantities and timing that they plan to use in the race. For example, if the aid stations are going

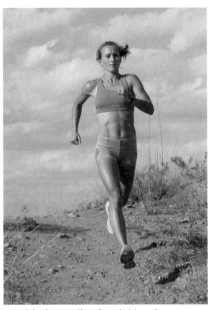

World-class miler Sarah Vaughn
Photo by 101 Degrees West

to be every 2 miles, then we should practice drinking the same energy drink, in the proper amount, every 2 miles during our longer training runs.

Marathon Hydration Logistics Example

The athlete in the Sweat Rate Test Example above determined that he or she needs to replenish fluids at a rate of about 32 ounces per hour in mild weather conditions. If the athlete plans to run a marathon in about 3:15 (which is about a 7:30 minute/mile pace) and has determined that the aid stations are spaced 2 miles apart, starting at the second mile marker, then he or she should practice drinking 8 ounces of fluid every 2 miles during long training runs.

Here is the calculation of how we determined the 8-ounce amount per aid station:

- A 7:30 minutes-per-mile pace = 8 miles per hour
- Aid stations are spaced every 2 miles, so the athlete will visit four aid

stations per hour (i.e., 8 miles per hour / 2 miles between aid stations = four aid stations per hour).

- Since the athlete needs to consume 32 ounces per hour, he or she needs to consume 8 ounces per aid station (i.e., 32 oz. / four aid stations = 8 oz. per aid station).

In the case of an athlete training for an Iron-distance triathlon, we usually suggest practicing with the energy drink the race will be offering for all long runs, and possibly long rides, depending on what he or she plans to do on race day. Remember, in the case of a triathlon, an athlete has the option of carrying his own bottles on his bike, which makes it much easier to stick with your preferred energy drink and not to have to use the one offered by the race, at least during the cycling portion.

For triathlons up to the half Iron-distance triathlon, one can pretty much carry all (or almost all) of one's own bottles. Due to the length of the full-distance Iron-distance race, this is not possible. Most Iron-distance races allow athletes to fill up a "special needs" bag with extra bottles, which the athlete can retrieve at about the halfway point on the bike course. These concessions vary from race to race, which makes it that much more important for an athlete to do a little research, at least a couple of months before the race, to find out what fluids they will offer, where they will offer them on the course, and what other rules apply. Then, the athlete needs to use this information to plan out an approach and then test that approach in training.

Iron-Distance Triathlon Bike Hydration Logistics Example

The athlete in the Sweat Rate Test example above determined that he or she needs to replenish fluids at a rate of about 32 ounces per hour. If the athlete is planning to complete the bike portion of an Iron-distance triathlon in about six hours, he or she has determined to practice completing a 24-ounce bottle of the energy drink every 45 minutes during long training rides.

Here is the calculation of how we determined the 45 minutes per bottle:

- 32 ounces per hour x 6 hours = 192 ounces for entire bike segment
- 192 ounces / 24-ounce bike bottles = 8 bottles required for entire bike course
- Since the athlete needs to consume 32 ounces per hour, he or she

needs to consume one bottle every 45 minutes (i.e., 6 hours / 8 bottles = 1 bottle every 45 minutes).

But what if we do it all correctly? We research the race website in advance and find out what the race fluid will be, and where and when it will be offered on the course, and we test it thoroughly in training, but we find that we still just don't like it, and/or our system doesn't seem to be able to tolerate it?

First, we suggest not making any kind of decision too quickly. If you try it out in training a couple of times and find that it doesn't appeal to you, give it another chance. Our bodies are trainable, even when it comes to our ability to consume fluids. While it may not appeal to us at first, if we continue to train with it, we may very well learn to like it, or at least get used to it. In certain races it is such an advantage to be able to use what the course offers the athletes that it's worth giving it some extra time to see if it can work for you.

But, if you do give it a fair shot in training (i.e., during all of your long runs, for four or five weeks) and it's still not working for you, then there are other hydration logistic options to consider.

Carrying Your Own Fluids

One popular option for marathons and ultras is to carry your own fluids on a fuel belt (sometimes also called a hydration belt). There are other popular fluid-carrying options, including handheld bottle-holders and camelbacks. Athletes typically train using one of these options, so it's easy for them to approach their racing in the same way.

There are some key issues to consider with this approach. First, carrying your own fluids adds weight, which means that you will spend some of your valuable energy transporting this weight. It's not a lot, but if you are going for a personal best time, you may want every bit of energy focused on propelling your body forward rather than carrying extra weight.

Second, carrying bottles adds bulk. This can have a negative impact on your running form and efficiency. Some athletes find the weight of the belt and fluids a distraction as they run.

Having said this, many of our coached athletes enjoy and prefer using a fuel belt. Most use a fuel belt every day in training and have become very comfortable doing so. Other advantages include not having to navigate through crowds at the aid stations, and the fact that flasks are more exacting and easier to drink from than paper cups.

If you think you would like to use a fuel/hydration belt, a handheld bottle-holder, or a camelback to carry your own fluids, practice with it for several weeks prior to your race, and make sure you are fully comfortable with it.

Hydrating at Aid Stations

Another option is to hydrate with water from the aid stations and make up the missed calories through some other means. We will cover the importance of consuming calories in the next chapter. For now, let's just stipulate that drinking water alone and consuming no calories during a long endurance event like a marathon, an ultra, or Iron-distance triathlon is not an option. One approach is to drink water at all of the aid stations to satisfy your hydration needs and then increase your fueling sources to compensate for the missed calories, sodium, and other electrolytes.

The following is an example of an athlete we coach who typically consumes about 28 ounces of his favorite energy drink every hour during his marathons, and also consumes a GU energy gel every 30 minutes. Since 28 ounces of his energy drink gives him 200 calories per hour, and his two GU energy gels give him 200 calories per hour, his usual total calories per hour are 400 calories. He can achieve the same targets with 28 ounces of water (0 calories) and a GU energy gel every 15 minutes (400 calories). Since he does not like any other energy drinks than his one favorite, and since he does like the GU energy gels, this strategy works well for him.

Another possible solution to the issue of not being able to use the energy drink offered by the race in a long-course triathlon, like an Iron-distance triathlon, is to use condensed bottles on the bike. A great example of this is an athlete we coach who typically covers a 112-mile Iron-distance bike course in a little less than five hours, and prefers a certain energy drink that he mixes from powder.

Since he completes a 20-ounce bottle every 40 minutes, he needs about eight bottles to complete a five-hour bike ride. Since carrying eight bottles on your bike is not a good option, it is possible to carry four bottles and then to pick up a second four in a special needs bag at about the halfway point.

While this is fine for some, he still feels that four bottles is more weight than he wants to carry on his bike in a race, and he prefers not to have to slow down or even stop to retrieve his special needs bag, so he utilizes the "condensed bottle strategy," mixing two bottles of his energy drink at four times the normal concentration. Therefore, each of the two bottles has four times the normal amount of calories and electrolytes. He then starts the race with these two mixed bottles, and takes six water bottles (one at a time) from aid stations along the course. He gradually mixes the two condensed bottles with the water in his aero drinking system as he goes.

There are several popular aero bottles and aero drinking systems available. What they all have in common is that they are hands-free, and are positioned right in front of the handlebars with a straw coming right up toward the rider's face. Typically, the rider only needs to lower his or her face slightly to draw fluids from the straw—a big plus, as it allows an athlete to remain in an aerodynamic position. The other main feature of the aero bottles is that they have some type of opening in the top to allow the rider to easily and efficiently refill while cycling.

By using condensed bottles, our athlete can have the same calories and the same fluids as normal, and he can do it with little outside assistance. In fact, if the athlete starts with the first bottle already mixed and in the aero bottle, then he only needs to take five bottles from aid stations along the way.

Normal drinking plan for this athlete:

- 8 bike bottles (20 oz. each) with 150 calories each = 160 ounces and 1,200 calories

Condensed-bottle plan for same athlete:

- 2 bike bottles (20 oz. each) with 600 calories each and 6 bike bottles (20 oz. each) of water = 160 ounces and 1,200 calories

Drinking from Cups while Racing

Many athletes have difficulty drinking from a cup during races. Cups at aid stations are common in most road races, the running portion of triathlons, and many other types of endurance races. The issue is that athletes often find that they spill much of the liquid while trying to drink it while in motion. Not

AN IRONFIT MOMENT

Changing Hydration Sources during Competition

Many athletes like to change their hydration sources during their competitions. Such changes are especially popular in Ultra Distance races, during which an athlete can grow very bored of the same drink hour after hour. Some athletes like to switch to de-fizzed cola toward the end of longer events to enjoy the benefits of the simple sugar and caffeine, as well as the flavor change. The practice is particularly popular in Iron-distance triathlons, when an athlete may drink water and an energy drink for the entire bike and the first half of the run, but then switch to de-fizzed cola in the last half of the marathon. Many Iron-distance triathlons offer de-fizzed cola at aid stations on the run course.

As with anything when it comes to racing, if you think you'd like to try it during your race, you should test it thoroughly in training. The last half of an Iron-distance marathon is not the time to say, "Gee, I think I'll try cola." But if you test it thoroughly in training and feel it benefits your performance, it may prove to be a good addition to your race-day hydration plan.

only is it then difficult to know how much you have consumed, but it's also uncomfortable to have sticky energy drink all over your hands and clothes.

What we suggest for most competitive athletes we work with is to practice good technique with this in training so that they are more proficient with it at the races. The best approach is to pinch the top of the cup together to reduce spillage and to form a sort of spout; then, pour the liquid into your mouth as swiftly and as neatly as possible. The only way to become competent is to practice this maneuver.

A great way to practice drinking from cups is to do it while running on a track. Set up your drinks on a table right next to the inside lane so that you can reach them from the track as you run by.

Another approach for drinking from cups during races is to walk for a few steps at the aid station. Most find it steadier and easier to drink down the contents of the cup while walking than while running. There are differing views on this method. We coach some athletes who are very skilled at going right into a quickly paced but smooth walk as soon as they take the cup; they consume it quickly and then get right back to running in only a few seconds. Many marathoners also use the run/walk approach popularized by the well-known athlete/coach Jeff Galloway. Drinking while in the walk portion works perfectly with this approach.

One additional approach is to take two cups at each station. If you spill most of the first one, or perhaps even drop it by mistake, you will still have a backup. Many athletes use this approach despite the fact that a lot of good energy drink gets wasted.

Now that we have discussed the above strategies and approaches for winning hydration, we will cover the importance of fueling in Chapter 7.

Powerful Fueling for Endurance Athletes

Fortune favors the brave.

—*Publius Terence*

It's amazing how the athletic benefit from consuming calories while training and competing has only recently become known and accepted. In fact, calorie consumption during athletic activity was often discouraged as a risk factor for cramping.

The revolution really took hold in the 1970s endurance sports community when Gatorade was introduced, and it became common knowledge that athletic performance improved with a fluid that contained calories, sodium, and other electrolytes.

The Importance of Fueling for Competition and Training

Today the benefit of consuming calories during endurance sports performance seems obvious. In our testing with coached athletes and our own training, it is very clear that the right amount and type of calories and fluids before and during exercise greatly improves performance. Furthermore, as the distance gets longer, the benefit of calories increases.

Of course, in the 1970s, Ultra Distance racing was not yet popular. Few endurance competitions lasted over 90 minutes, and even the marathon, which began to gain in popularity during the 1970s, was still only considered possible for a few superathletes.

Today we understand that water alone won't do it for longer competitions. Without sufficient calories beyond a certain point, the dreaded "bonk" is unavoidable. The "bonk" is that terrible feeling when you run out of energy and feel completely flat. As the saying goes, "It feels like you are trying to run with a piano on your back."

AN IRONFIT MOMENT

Plenty has been written and discussed in endurance sports circles regarding the important role played by calories, carbohydrates, protein, fat, sodium, and electrolytes. Surprisingly, however, we often find that most endurance athletes don't know what these things are.

Here's a quick and to-the-point explanation:

Calories, carbohydrates, proteins, and fats: A calorie is a basic unit of energy. When a certain food is said to have 100 calories, it simply means that it contains 100 units of energy. Carbohydrates and proteins have about 4 calories per gram, while fat has about 9 calories per gram.

Electrolytes and sodium: Common examples of electrolytes are sodium, potassium, and chloride. Our cells need electrolytes in order to function properly. Some electrolytes, like sodium, can be lost through exercise and perspiration.

The 75-Minute Fueling Guideline

In our own testing, we find that if we are properly fueled and hydrated prior to the start of a training session, our performance in that training session can be just as good if we're hydrating with plain water as it is if we're hydrating with water plus some additional calorie source, through about 75 minutes. After 75 minutes, however, our performance starts to deteriorate without adding calories. We need fuel, and when we say fuel, we mean calories.

While we encourage our coached athletes to be well fueled and hydrated before they start a training session, once they begin their workouts, we suggest they hydrate with just straight water for sessions of up to 75 minutes. For workouts longer than 75 minutes, we suggest they begin fueling along with their hydration right from the start. We call this the 75-minute fueling guideline.

For your 60-minute run, you may just consume water. For your 90-minute, you need to consume either an energy drink, or water combined with some other calorie source.

Aerobic vs. Anaerobic Systems

It is our goal not to get overly technical in this book. After having coached athletes for many years, we know that heavy nutritional and exercise science are not what they want. Most athletes want helpful information that they can take with them and put right to work. A lot of technical lingo is distracting. But we need to have a basic conversation about energy systems in order to really understand what we need to do.

Our energy systems include the aerobic energy system, which is fueled primarily by utilizing oxygen and stored fat, and the anaerobic energy system, which is fueled primarily by utilizing stored sugar (glycogen). The aerobic energy system is associated more with moderate intensities of athletic activity, while anaerobic is associated with high intensities of activity.

Let's start with some basic definitions:

- Aerobic energy system: An energy system that primarily utilizes oxygen and stored fat to power physical activity. This system can support activity for prolonged periods, as stored fat and oxygen are available in almost endless supply. Even a highly trained athlete with body fat percentages in the single digits has more than enough stored fat for several Ultra Distance races back to back.
- Anaerobic energy system: An energy system that primarily utilizes glycogen (stored sugar) to power physical activity. This system can support activity for relatively short periods of time, as the body stores sugar in relatively small quantities.

One of the key points to understand is that both systems are always working; the ratio at which we utilize the two systems changes as the intensity of the activity changes, but they are both always contributing to the athlete's physical movements. At low to moderate levels of activity, we are relying more on the aerobic system, and therefore more on oxygen and body fat to fuel our activity.

As the intensity increases, however, the ratio shifts, and we start relying more and more on anaerobic energy. We start burning more of the body's stored glycogen to fuel our activity.

Here's the next key point to understand: While the aerobic system has an almost infinite source of fuel (i.e., oxygen and the body's stored fat), the anaerobic system's fuel—stored sugar (glycogen)—is held by the body in relatively limited quantities.

Low storage is why higher-intensity activity cannot be maintained for a long period. Eventually the glycogen runs out, and we experience the "bonk." Avoiding the bonk and maximizing our training and racing requires us not only to target the proper level of intensity, but also to fuel properly in order to sustain the energy level necessary to maximize our performance.

Most athletes and even some coached athletes don't fully grasp that we are always using both systems all of the time. Again, it's just the usage ratio of the two that changes. Even when we are training at a fairly moderate level and relying mostly on our aerobic system, we are still relying somewhat on our anaerobic system. Therefore, we are still using the body's glycogen stores. While these stores are usually enough to carry us through a 75-minute workout, after that point, our glycogen stores are often too low to support our activity, meaning our performance will suffer. Thus, we need to fuel with calories during workouts and races that will last longer than about 75 minutes.

Calories Needed Before Training

Many athletes make the mistake of starting their training sessions with insufficient fueling. They may be rushed for time, or they may mistakenly think that they can "catch up" on fueling as they go.

In a well-designed training plan, every training session is an opportunity to become stronger and faster. To maximize the benefits of a specific training session, we need to be properly energized and focused. Starting the session with a low energy level will lower the potential benefit of the session, and often leave the athlete feeling flat and discouraged.

We often hear complaints from athletes who are concerned about a bad workout session. They felt flat, unable to raise their heart rates up into the range prescribed for the workout. We typically ask two questions of an athlete in this situation: What, and how much, did he or she hydrate and fuel with in the hours leading up to the workout? While lack of sleep and high stress levels are also common culprits, more often than not we find that the athlete was underhydrated, underfueled, or both. To maximize the benefit of our training, we always need to be properly fueled and hydrated right at the start.

AN IRONFIT MOMENT

Pre-Training Session Fueling and Hydration Example

Don typically swims in our local Masters Swimming program three times a week. The Friday-morning session starts at the unpleasant hour of 5:45 a.m. To feel properly fueled and hydrated for this particular workout, Don typically has the following pre-swim routine:

- Wakes at 4:45 a.m. (one hour before his swim).
- Drinks 12 ounces of water with a PowerBar (240 calories).
- Drinks an 8-ounce coffee.
- Dresses for swimming.
- While driving to the pool, Don consumes a GU energy gel (100 calories) and 12 ounces of energy drink (90 calories).
- Enters the pool at 5:45 a. m.

Total Pre-Workout Fluids and Calories:

- Total Fluids = 32 ounces
- Total Calories = 430

To many athletes, these totals may seem high, but this type of approach has Don feeling awake and energized at the start of this 65- to 75-minute swim, and Don continues to feel a strong energy level throughout, despite burning between 900 and 1,000 calories. The key for most athletes is to start small and then gradually see what amounts and types of fueling and hydration best prepare you for your workout.

In Chapter 8, we will present several pre-training and pre-race fueling routines to help you identify your optimal fueling strategy.

Calories Needed during Training and Competition

In general we find that most athletes are too light on their fueling during training and competition. As per the 75-minute guideline we discussed earlier, it's usually not necessary to fuel at all during training sessions of 75 minutes or less, especially if you are properly fueled before you begin, but for longer training sessions and competitions, fueling is very important.

Depending on the specific activity and the intensity of that activity, an athlete can expend hundreds and hundreds of calories per hour. An experienced Iron-distance triathlete will easily burn 800 to 1,000 calories per hour. If it takes the athlete ten hours to complete the race, that equates to 8,000 to 10,000 calories. It's not necessary to replace all of those calories, but the athlete does need to replace a good deal of them.

You can maximize your performance by replacing between one-third and one-half of the calories expended during longer training sessions and races. The longer the competition, typically the more important it is to be on the higher end of that 33 to 50 percent range. Every athlete is unique, and different things work for different people, but most athletes will benefit from working within this targeted range.

We have coached many Iron-distance triathletes and ultra-marathoners who benefited from a fueling plan that replaced as many as 500 or more calories per hour. It makes sense: For an elite athlete who is burning up to about 1,000 calories per hour, 500 calories represents calorie replacement of about 50 percent. For shorter races—say, an Olympic-distance triathlon—this same athlete may perform better with only about 350 calories per hour. That intake puts the athlete closer to 33 percent, which is the lower end of the range.

As important as the amount of calories is the timing of the calorie intake. We want to consume them as evenly as possible. If our plan is for 350 calories per hour, we want to consume those 350 calories in small portions spread evenly over the hour. Furthermore, we want each hour to be pretty much the same. We don't want to have 200 calories in one hour and 500 calories in another and feel that we are fine simply because we are still averaging our targeted amount of 350 calories. We want to come as close to our target as possible in each and every hour.

We recall a conversation on this topic we had many years ago with Iron-distance and international-distance world champion Karen Smyers. We were talking about how we wanted to consume our calories as evenly as possible for optimal performance. Karen joked that in the future they would probably have some sort of IV-drip technology system set up on your bike that would be able to gradually provide you with the perfect level of calories, as evenly as possible, over the course of your race. While just a joke, this is a good visualization for the important point here. We want to take in just the right amount of fuel at a very even and constant rate. The better we are at mimicking this approach, the better we will be at maintaining a consistent energy level.

The biggest mistake we can make with our fueling is to forget to eat for a long period of time and then try to play catch-up on calories. This rarely ever works. We have seen this issue with many first-time Iron-distance athletes and marathoners. They have a well-thought-out fueling plan before the race, but then in the excitement of the big day, they forget or fall behind on their plan. Falling behind on fuel will make a long day that much longer.

Precise fueling is especially important in a race like the Iron-distance triathlon, which starts with a swim. There are no opportunities to consume calories while swimming. The race itself is designed in such a way as to easily put you in a calorie deficit right from the start.

For example, say that a particular first-time Iron-distance triathlete successfully completes the swim in 75 minutes, but then is so excited about his big race that he forgets to start fueling for the first 45 minutes of the bike. This athlete has already gone two hours without any calories, and is in serious trouble before the day has barely begun.

The best way to stick with your plan is to "eat on the clock." We encourage our coached athletes to start their chrono watch as soon as they mount their bike, and from that point on, let the clock tell them when to eat and drink. Some athletes like to set the beeper on their watch to give them a reminder.

In Chapter 8 we will provide examples of successful fueling and hydration plans, and offer suggestions to help you put together an optimal fueling and hydration routine for racing success.

Calories Needed after Training and Competition

While our calorie needs are sometimes overlooked, or at least given improperly low priority, at no time are they more ignored than after training and racing.

There is a short period of time, usually about 45 minutes following our training sessions and races, during which we have an opportunity to jump-start our recovery. If we are able to consume the proper amount of

AN IRONFIT MOMENT

An elite triathlete we coach has a simple Iron-distance fueling and hydration routine of consuming an energy gel every 25 minutes and completing a 20-ounce bike bottle of energy drink every 35 minutes. To make this easier, and to give himself something to mentally focus on during the race, he writes the times by which he needs to complete each bottle on a piece of white medical tape, and the exact times at which he needs to consume a gel on another piece of white medical tape. He then attaches both pieces of tape to his bike handlebars, in clear view.

The one that provides drinking times looks something like this:

0:35	2:55
1:10	3:30
1:45	4:05
2:20	4:40

His first bottle needs to be completed within the first 35 minutes. The next bottle needs to be completed by the time of 1 hour and 10 minutes. And so on.

The one that provides energy gel times looks something like this:

0:25	2:55
0:50	3:20
1:15	3:45
1:40	4:10
2:05	4:35
2:30	

His first gel needs to be consumed at 25 minutes, the next one at 50 minutes—and so on.

In addition to keeping his fueling and hydration plan right on schedule, he also likes how this approach keeps him mentally focused during the race. After he either consumes a gel or completes a bottle, he then turns his focus to the next time on his chart. This helps both to segment the race for him and to stay mentally dialed in to his race plan.

carbohydrates and protein during this period, along with proper hydration, we are giving our body what it needs right when it needs it. We will not only help to repair the damage done during training and racing, but we will also start the process of building back even stronger. In addition, it helps our body to start replenishing its levels of stored glycogen. This important glycogen-level replacement process can take twenty hours or more, depending on the athlete and the situation.

There is something very special about our post-workout refueling opportunity. Some call it the "45-minute window." If we are able to start refueling right away with the proper amounts of carbohydrates and protein, our bodies are much more able to fully replenish our glycogen levels by the next day's workout. In other words, not only did we have a great workout today, but now we've set ourselves up for having another great and productive workout tomorrow.

If, on the other hand, we skip or forget to refuel properly during the 45-minute window, we greatly lessen the chances that our bodies will be as fully recovered and prepared for the next day's workout.

That's not such a big deal, right? Well, if you miss the 45-minute window on a fairly regular basis, a couple very negative trends develop.

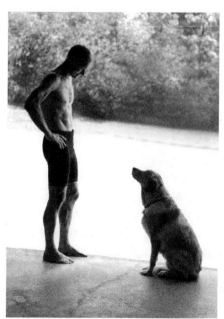

First, you do not feel as energized as you need to be before the next workout. Typically this is evident by your mental attitude. You will not be as excited and focused for your workout, and will feel as though you are forcing yourself to train.

Second, if you have planned a higher-intensity workout, then you may find it unusually difficult to push yourself to that level, and this usually results in lower training heart rates than what you are trying to achieve.

Elite 50-plus endurance athlete
Jeff Kellogg with Kula
Photo by Lynn Kellogg/
www.trilifephotos.com

Finally, if you make it a habit to skip the 45-minute window, you risk a general overall feeling of fatigue. Some describe it as a "burnt-out" feeling. The fatigue of one day just rolls right into the next, and a long period of feeling run-down ensues. Now you not only risk losing the benefits of training, but you can also suffer injury and illness.

In Chapter 8, we will present several post-training and post-race fueling routines for your consideration.

"You Need a Hearty Breakfast!"

Back when Don was a high school track athlete, there was very little attention given to hydration, let alone fueling. Don doesn't even recall such concepts being commonly discussed between athletes and coaches. Instead, they ate and drank what they wanted and showed up to track practice and started running. It rarely ever occurred to anyone that how they felt and performed in practice, let alone in races, had very much to do with what they ate or drank each day.

On the rare occasion when thought was given to an endurance athlete's nutrition, it was usually misguided and based on some old flawed belief or half-truth, like, "Meat is protein and protein builds muscle. So that's what athletes need to eat!"

Don likes to tell the story about when his dad insisted that he have a "good hearty breakfast" one Saturday morning when he was heading out to a track meet. He sat Don down and kindly cooked him a big breakfast of fried Spam and eggs, buttered toast, and a tall glass of whole milk. He meant well, and was confident that this was the kind of breakfast needed before athletic competition.

As discussed earlier, both protein and fat play an important role in an endurance athlete's diet. But the types of protein and fat sources and the timing of the consumption is equally important. Carbohydrates are the most easily digestible energy source for most athletes, and provide the quickest energy response. The closer we are to the time of the race or training session, the more our calorie sources should lean toward simple carbohydrates.

While the flaws in Don's father's approach are clear to Don today, they weren't then. You would think Don might have gotten a clue when during the final lap of the mile race he found himself slowing from first to fourth place and throwing up just as he crossed the finish line. Oh well, some of us just have to learn the hard way.

The funny thing is that if all Don had consumed before that race was a bottle of cola and a candy bar, he would have been much better prepared to race. It sounds crazy, but junk food like cola and candy would have served him much better than a hearty breakfast. Of course, we're not recommending a cola-and-candy pre-race meal; there are much better options out there!

Determining Your Optimal Fueling Sources

Selecting the fueling sources that are best for you is very important. Many athletes tend to make this decision based on an advertisement they may have read about the latest "super fuel," or what some famous professional triathlete is using. Every such athlete is making another big rookie mistake.

The best way to determine the calorie sources that work for you is to test and experiment frequently in training, especially in your longer training sessions, which tend to best simulate race-day conditions.

There are plenty of great resources in this book to help you determine the best fueling plan for you, including several plans in Chapter 8 with which you can experiment during training.

Fueling Logistics

A very important but often overlooked aspect of proper fueling is how you plan logistically to get your fuel sources. You can have the best fueling plan in the world, but it will do you no good unless it's easy to accomplish on race day. Having the right type of fuel, in the right amount, available to you at the right time, does not just happen; it takes careful planning and practice.

In general, we have three possibilities available to us. We can either 1) carry our fuel, 2) get it from aid stations on the course, or 3) do a combination of the two. There are pros and cons to each alternative.

The biggest advantage of using the aid stations is that you don't have to bother carrying your fuel sources; someone at the aid station will literally hand it to you as you go by. The disadvantages with aid stations are numerous—a lot can (and will) go wrong. The well-intentioned volunteers may drop something as they give it to you, requiring you to stop and retrieve it, or they may hand you the wrong item. Aid stations also often run out of items—usually the exact item you want.

If you are a back-of-the-pack competitor, you are very likely to experience situations where aid stations will run out of exactly what you want. If you are a middle-of-the-pack competitor, you will often find that the aid stations are crowded when you get there, and you have difficulty finding what you want, or finding a volunteer who can help you. Such scenarios can be hugely frustrating as the seconds tick by and you have your sights set on a new personal record performance.

If you are a front-of-the-pack competitor, you may encounter aid stations that are not ready for you. Back in Don's younger years he had the good fortune to find himself in the lead on the marathon run in the Vineman Triathlon (Iron-distance) in Santa Rosa, California. As he approached one of the early aid stations on the run course, he yelled ahead, "Cola!" One of the volunteers replied "Cola?" and looked confused, as if to say, "Now let's see, where can I find that cola?" It didn't look like Don was going to get his cola, until, at the very last second, a young boy who was there volunteering with his family pulled an unopened 2-liter bottle of warm cola out of a bag he found behind the table and handed it to Don. "Thanks, buddy!" Don said, as he saw how hard the kid was working, adding, "But I just changed my mind—I'm going to grab one of these cups of energy drink instead. Keep up the great work!"

Most races will announce in advance on their website what foods and drinks they will be offering on the course, as well as where on the course the aid stations will be located. Considering this information is a very good place to start before putting your plan together.

Carbohydrate Loading

We frequently get asked about carbohydrate loading, and whether or not it's something athletes should consider. The first thing to address is all the confusion that exists over what exactly is meant by this term. To most athletes today, it means eating a lot of carbohydrate-rich foods the night before the race, usually in the form of a big pasta dinner.

Technically, true carbohydrate loading addresses the theory that if you deplete your body of carbohydrates for a period of time (usually a few days) by eating a low-carbohydrate diet, you can then set your body up to store more carbohydrates than usual when you switch to a diet rich in carbohydrates for a period of time (usually a few days) just prior to the race. True carbohydrate loading also includes a hard training session right before the athlete begins the few days of low-carbohydrate eating, which is believed to further enhance the depletion process.

Carbohydrates are stored as glycogen, which, as discussed earlier in this chapter, is a key element for endurance sports success. The theory goes that if you starve yourself from carbohydrates, you then increase your ability to store more glycogen once you switch back to a diet heavy in carbohydrates.

A simple example of a carbohydrate-loading approach would be to start with a hard training session on the weekend before your big race. Then, begin eating a diet very low in carbohydrates right through Tuesday of a Saturday race week. Then, switch to eating a diet very rich in carbohydrates from Wednesday to Friday. If the approach works, you will have an extra high level of glycogen for your Saturday race.

There are pros and cons to this approach, of course. It may be worth considering for some athletes, but it may not be for others.

One of the risks is that an athlete eating foods that he or she is not used to will throw off mind and body during the week before the race. Our bodies get used to our routines, especially the foods we consume, and it's a risk to throw your body a curveball right before the big day. Different foods may make you feel physically flat, or worse yet, they may cause gastrointestinal distress (G-I) distress, which is definitely not what we want to be dealing with on race-day morning.

In general, it's risky to do anything new or to change your routine in the week prior to a race. Race week is not the time to test anything. Unless you are willing to try a carbohydrate-loading approach at least a couple of times during training to practice it, we don't suggest trying it for the first time before a big race. In fact, one of the most common categories of rookie mistakes is making last-minute changes in some key element before a race.

Another risk to carbohydrate loading is catching a cold or some other illness right before the race. Over the years, we have noticed an increased occurrence of unwellness in athletes attempting a carbo-loading process, which potentially can lower your immunity.

So, while we would not discourage you from testing a true carbo-loading approach in training to see if it's something that works for you, what we are more comfortable suggesting is for athletes to consider an approach of "topping off your glycogen."

Instead of going through the carbohydrate-depletion phase discussed above, simply stick with your normal diet at the start of race week. Once you enter the last forty-eight to seventy-two hours before the race, start to switch your calorie sources over to more carbohydrate-rich foods (preferably low in fiber). Don't try new carbohydrate sources at this point, however; stick with ones that you are used to in your regular diet. All we will be doing here is increasing the percentage of your diet made up of your familiar carbohydrates.

This approach is less risky than carbohydrate loading. Not only will you probably feel better during race week, but, more importantly, you will feel energized and strong on race-day morning when you step up to the starting line.

Along with carbohydrates, it's also helpful for endurance athletes (especially "salty sweaters") to increase their sodium intake in the days leading up to a major race. A sodium boost can be accomplished by slightly increasing the amount of salt consumed in food. A great carbohydrate-rich food we like to snack on in the last forty-eight to seventy-two hours before a race is pretzels. Not only will pretzels help to top off your glycogen stores, but they will also boost your sodium levels as well.

Should You Include Caffeine in Your Plan?

The benefits of moderate levels of caffeine on endurance sports performance are well documented. We have also seen clear evidence of it in our own training and racing, as well as with many of our coached athletes over the years.

If you feel you would like to see if caffeine works for you in your racing, and your doctor has specifically cleared you to consume caffeine, our suggestion is to play it safe and start with only modest amounts. See how it makes you feel and perform in training, and then, through proper testing, determine the optimal levels for you. Many athletes find that it helps, but others report that it made them feel nervous and jittery. If the latter is true for you, don't do it; it's not for you.

The two most common ways to consume caffeine for training and racing purposes are to simply drink a caffeinated beverage before you start, and/or

AN IRONFIT MOMENT

A Word on Salt and Electrolyte Tablets

We are frequently asked by athletes if they should take salt tablets to improve their racing performance. As presented earlier in this chapter, our cells need electrolytes to function properly. Sodium (salt) is an important electrolyte, and it can be lost through exercise and perspiration.

Because of this, many athletes take a variety of salt and electrolyte tablets in the hope of improving their performance. While salt and electrolyte tablets can be beneficial for some athletes, what we tend to find is that many athletes quickly jump to taking salt tablets before first properly addressing their fueling and hydration needs. The majority of athletes can receive the electrolytes they need through a proper fueling and hydration routine, and adding salt tablets on top of this may just be overkill, while also adding another layer of complication.

Having said this, we have also discussed the risks of hyponatremia (diluted sodium levels) in the previous chapter. So, proper sodium levels are something all endurance athletes should take seriously and address proactively—especially those who are "salty sweaters."

Our suggestion for most athletes is first to use all of the approaches and suggestions in this book, including our suggested Sweat Rate Test protocol, to build your optimal fueling and hydration plan. Consider trying to get all of your sodium from your fueling and hydration sources.

For example, some energy drinks have up to 200 milligrams of sodium per 8 ounces, and some energy gels have from 20 to over 100 milligrams per serving. For most athletes, these are the most convenient ways to consume their proper amount of sodium. Test these options thoroughly in training and see what methods and amounts work best for you. Then, if you would like to experiment with adding salt or electrolyte tablets to the mix, first clear it with your doctor, and then safely test it in training, starting with very modest, safe levels. (Note: When taking salt or electrolyte tablets, always do so with water.)

Remember, salt and electrolyte tablets may help, but they are not a replacement for a proper fueling and hydration routine.

to consume energy gels with caffeine while you train or race. GU Energy has gels with and without caffeine, as well as those with a double amount of caffeine. Most other energy gel companies have both caffeinated and non-caffeinated products. Again, start with a very modest level and be safe.

There are various strategies for maximizing the benefit of caffeine on race day. One popular approach is to stop consuming all forms of caffeine about ten days prior to the race. Then, on race-day morning, have your regular coffee or caffeinated gel. Supposedly you will derive a greater benefit than if you had been drinking your normal amount of caffeine all along. Personally, we have tried this strategy and did not see any increased benefit to our performance, although some athletes we know say that it works for them.

The bottom line is this: Caffeine in the proper moderate amount does have a small positive impact on the performance of some athletes. The key is to play it safe, get cleared by your doctor, and then proceed with moderation.

CHAPTER 8

Fueling and Hydration Plans for Training and Competition

Strength does not come from physical
capacity. It comes from an indomitable will.

—Gandhi

In the previous two chapters we discussed the fundamentals and importance of proper fueling and hydration before, during, and after endurance sports racing and training. We also discussed race fueling and hydration logistics, and included some examples of actual fueling and hydration plans for specific situations. In this chapter, we will present the full and complete fueling and hydration routines for eight experienced and accomplished athletes.

These plans are the real deal, not the result of some recent fad or marketing hype. The plans were developed and fine-tuned over years of trial and error by eight exceptional athletes competing in the world's most grueling and challenging endurance sports competitions. The athletes used these plans because they work, and have allowed them to accomplish amazing racing results.

As we have found through our many years of coaching all types of endurance athletes, some busy, time-crunched athletes may be interested in the rationale behind everything, but what they all really want is clear direction on what to do. Athletes don't want to be educated on the science of fueling and hydration but then be left to put together a plan on their own. We can hear their voices in our heads right now: "I'm so busy, Coach. Can you just tell me what I should eat and drink during my race?"

Well, if you feel this way, then this chapter is for you. We have presented eight complete fueling and hydration plans for you to consider and try for yourself. Not only do these plans cover before, during, and after training and racing, but they also consider several different types and distances of endurance sports and many different athlete preferences, as well.

Every athlete is unique, and following these plans may not be the best choice for you. You will only know this for sure by putting them to the test in training and then fine-tuning them based on your results. Still, these plans contain many cutting-edge ideas and approaches that you can immediately start to use in your own training and racing.

Fuel and Hydrate Like the Experienced Ones

In this section we will present the complete fueling and hydration plans for the following eight experienced and accomplished endurance athletes:

1. Scott Boyles
2. Kellie Brown
3. Scott Gac
4. Peter Hyland
5. Dave Mantle
6. Russ O'Hara
7. Greg Perangelo
8. Peter Turek

The important thing to keep in mind is that these athletes have all raced at a high level for many years, and they've battle-tested and honed their fueling and hydration plans over this time. Most of these athletes started training and racing at lower levels of fueling and hydration, but they learned early on that in order to maximize their performance, they needed to increase their fueling and hydration intake. Over time they worked on training their bodies to gradually take in more, and eventually they found their optimal levels. It took discipline, consistency, and patience. While every athlete is different, we encourage you to consider the wisdom in their approaches and put them to good use.

Before we get into the details of each of the eight athletes' plans, the following is a summary of some of the key statistics from their pre-race and race fueling and hydration plans:

Eight Athletes' Pre-Race Fueling and Hydration Statistics

Fluid ounces consumed: 45 to 72 oz. (range)
Fluid ounces (oz.) to body weight (lbs.) ratio: 0.36 (average); 0.28 to 0.43 (range)

Calories consumed: 690 to 1,212 (range)
Calories to body weight (lbs.) ratio: 6.6 (average); 5.7 to 7.3 (range)

Nutritional ratio (average): 76% carbohydrates, 12% protein, and 12% fat

---

Note: Some of the athletes modify their plans based on the time it takes them to complete the race. For example, some athletes have a slightly different plan for shorter races versus longer races. For athletes with these types of multilevel plans, the details from their "long plan" are included in the above statistics for comparative purposes.

The pre-race fluid consumption for the eight athletes ranges from 45 to 72 ounces. What this means is that from the time they wake up on race-day morning until the time the gun goes off a few hours later, each of these athletes usually consumes an amount of fluid within this range.

Since athletes vary in body weight, we like to apply a simple ratio of ounces of fluid to pounds of body weight to help get a better apples-to-apples comparison of one athlete to another. As you can see in the statistics above, the average for the athletes was 0.36 ounces of fluid per pound of body weight, and all of the athletes fell into a range of 0.28 to 0.43. This simply means that all eight of these athletes consume an amount between 0.28 and 0.43 ounces of fluid per pound of body weight.

This ratio range can be a valuable piece of information as you put together your own personal plan. While all athletes are different, it is helpful to consider whether or not your pre-race hydration falls into the 0.28 to 0.43 range of these experienced athletes.

The pre-race calorie consumption for the eight athletes ranges from 690 to 1,212 calories. This means that from the time they wake up on race-day morning until the time the gun goes off a few hours later, each of these athletes usually consumes an amount of calories within this range.

To account for differences in body weight, we like to apply a ratio of the number of calories consumed to the number of pounds of body weight. As you can see in the statistics above, the average ratio for the group is 6.6

calories per pound of body weight, and the range of ratios for the athletes is 5.7 to 7.3. What this simply means is that on average, for each pound of body weight, the athletes consume 6.6 calories before the race.

This ratio range can also be a valuable piece of information as you plan your own pre-race fueling plan. While all athletes differ somewhat, it may be helpful to consider a pre-race calorie amount within the range of these eight experienced athletes.

Finally, the statistics above include the average nutritional breakdown for the eight athletes as being 76 percent carbohydrates, 12 percent protein, and 12 percent fat. As we will see in the actual presentation of each athlete's plan, most tended to be fairly close to these averages. So, this is another helpful guideline to use as you develop your own fueling and hydration routine.

Now that we have taken an overall look at the pre-race fueling and hydration plan statistics, we will take a similar look at the statistics for the eight athletes' actual race fueling plans.

Eight Athletes' Race Fueling and Hydration Statistics

Fluid ounces consumed per hour: 24 to 43 oz. (range)
Fluid (oz.) per hour to body weight (lbs.) ratio: 0.20 (average); 0.15 to 0.24 (range)

Calories per hour: 270 to 537 (range)
Calories to body weight (lbs.) ratio: 2.6 (average); 1.7 to 3.3 (range)

Nutritional ratio (range): 93 to 100% carbohydrates, 0 to 5 % protein, and 0 to 2% fat.

Note: Some of the athletes modify their plans based on the time it takes them to complete the race. For example, some athletes have a slightly different plan for shorter races versus longer races. For athletes with these types of multilevel plans, the details from their "long plan" are included in the above statistics for comparative purposes.

Once racing, the eight athletes all consume an amount of fluid in the range of 24 to 43 ounces per hour. To again account for differences in body weight, we have also calculated their ratios of fluid ounces consumed to body weight in pounds. The average was about 0.20 ounces per pound, and the athletes all fell within a range of 0.15 to 0.24.

Also recall that earlier in this book we introduced our suggested Sweat Rate Test protocol. The Sweat Rate Test should be the first step you take in determining your hydration needs for racing, while the range of ratios from these experienced athletes above provides an additional helpful guideline to consider as you fine-tune your plan.

The calories consumed per hour range from 270 to 537, and on average the athletes consumed 2.6 calories for every pound of body weight, with a range of 1.7 to 3.3. So, this is another good piece of information to take into account when perfecting your own plan.

Earlier in this book we discussed that you should also consider replacing your calories during competitions, especially longer competitions, at a rate of 33 percent to 50 percent. So this guideline, combined with the above 1.7 to 3.3 ratio ranges of calories to body weight, can really help you nail down exactly what your calorie replacement targets should be.

Finally, five of the eight athletes consumed 100 percent carbohydrates during their competitions. Many athletes find they perform better with some protein and fat. We will touch more on the topic of using fats and protein during racing later in this chapter.

We will now introduce our eight athletes and their specific fueling and hydration plans.

1. Endurance Athlete: Scott Boyles

Scott Boyles has raced competitively for several years, and focuses primarily on all triathlon distances up to Iron-distance, and all road-racing distances up to the full marathon. Scott frequently wins or places in his age group at all distances. Among his many accomplishments, Scott has recorded multiple Iron-distance times under 9:50. Scott's height is 5 feet, 10 inches, and he races at about 150 pounds.

Scott Boyles's Pre-Race Fueling and Hydration Routine

For longer races like the Iron-distance triathlon, Scott wakes up at least three hours before the start and consumes three PowerBars (720 calories; about 70% carbohydrates, 15% fat, and 15% protein) with 8 ounces of tea. From that point up until the start of the race, Scott gradually sips another 8 ounces of tea, 22 ounces of coconut water (120 calories, about 97% carbohydrates, 0% fat, and 3% protein), and 20 ounces of water with a Nuun electrolyte tablet (6 calories, all carbohydrates). Then, 10 minutes before the start, Scott consumes one GU Roctane energy gel (100 calories, all carbohydrates).

Scott Boyles's Pre-Race Fueling and Hydration Statistics (Approx.)

Fluid ounces consumed: 58 oz.
Fluid (oz.) to body weight (lbs.) ratio: 0.39

Calories consumed: 946
Calories to body weight (lbs.) ratio: 6.3

Nutritional ratios: 74% carbohydrates, 15% protein, and 11% fat

---

Scott Boyles's Race Fueling and Hydration Routine

For longer competitions like the Iron-distance triathlon, Scott consumes a GU Roctane energy gel (100 calories, all carbohydrates) as soon as he settles in on his bike, and then another gel every 30 minutes thereafter until crossing the finish line on the run. Scott rotates his energy gels on the bike in a sequence where the first is 100 percent carbohydrates with no caffeine, the second is 100 percent carbohydrates with caffeine, and the third has no caffeine, but does have 5 grams of protein. After years of trial and error, Scott finds this combination works best for him. On the bike Scott very evenly hydrates with 24 ounces of energy drink per hour (180 calories, all carbohydrates), and then targets the same even amount on the run both using his fuel belt and taking cups at aid stations.

Scott Boyles's Race Fueling and Hydration Statistics (Approx.)

Fluid ounces consumed per hour: 24 oz.
Fluid (oz.) per hour as a percentage of body weight (lbs.): 0.16

Calories per hour: 380
Calories per hour to body weight (lbs.) ratio: 2.5

Nutritional ratios: 95% carbohydrates, 5% protein, 0% fat

Scott Boyles's Pre-Training Fueling and Hydration Routine

Scott begins his regular weekday bike and run sessions in the early morning, and typically drinks 8 to 16 ounces of tea before bike sessions, and 4 to 8 ounces before run sessions. Scott's swims are typically in the early afternoon, and since they are fairly soon after lunchtime, he doesn't usually eat before, but if on occasion he feels like he needs a little extra energy, he will usually eat half of a small box of raisins. Scott drinks water during all of his shorter training sessions, and during his longer training sessions of over 75 minutes, he consumes energy drinks and energy gels to practice his race fueling and hydration routine.

Scott Boyles's Post-Training Fueling and Hydration Routine

Immediately after all regular training sessions, Scott consumes his own homemade 350-calorie recovery shake, which contains coconut water, Recoverite, Ultragen, whey protein, and blueberries. The shake has a ratio of approximately 4 to 1 carbohydrates to protein. Scott finds that this mixture speeds his recovery and prepares him well for his next training session.

2. Endurance Athlete: Kellie Brown

Kellie Brown has raced competitively for more than ten years. She focuses primarily on triathlons up to and including the full Iron-distance, and road races up to and including the marathon. Kellie frequently wins or places in her age group at all distances, and among her many accomplishments she has qualified for and raced the Boston Marathon multiple times. Kellie's height is 5 feet, 5 inches, and she races at about 115 pounds.

Kellie Brown's Pre-Race Fueling and Hydration Routine

Kellie wakes up at least three hours before the start and immediately consumes 8 ounces of either Boost or Ensure nutrition drink (250 calories, about 65% carbohydrates, 14% protein, and 21% fat). Then, at about two hours before the race, Kellie has a second meal, including ⅓ cup of oatmeal (100 calories; about 66% carbohydrates, 12% protein, and 22% fat) with 6 ounces of skim milk (67 calories; about 60% carbohydrates and 40% protein), plus 14 ounces of coffee with cream (90 calories; about 15% carbohydrates, 10%

protein, and 75% fat). From this point until the start of the race, Kellie gradually consumes 15 ounces of water. If the start is delayed, or if she was not able to complete all of the above calorie sources as planned, Kellie will consume an energy gel (100 calories; all carbohydrates) 15 minutes before the start. For longer races of about five hours or more (e.g., half and full Iron-distance triathlons), Kellie consumes a second 8 ounces of Boost or Ensure nutrition drink (250 calories; about 65% carbohydrates, 24% protein, and 21% fat) instead of the oatmeal in the second meal.

Kellie Brown's Pre-Race (Races of Five Hours or More) Fueling and Hydration Statistics (Approx.)

Fluid ounces consumed: 45 oz.
Fluid (oz.) to body weight (lbs.) ratio: 0.39

Calories consumed: 690
Calories to body weight (lbs.) ratio: 6.0

Nutritional ratios: 57 to 63% carbohydrates, 12 to 14% protein, and 25 to 29% fat

---

Kellie Brown's Race Fueling and Hydration Routine

Iron-Distance Triathlon: Kellie has her first caffeinated energy gel (100 calories, all carbohydrates) 15 minutes into the bike leg, and then takes one every 30 minutes thereafter. She drinks some water with each energy gel, but otherwise she targets 24 ounces of Gatorade or Perform energy drink per hour on the bike leg. Once on the run, Kellie follows a very similar routine to her marathon routine below, which includes a target of up to five caffeinated GU Roctane energy gels consumed evenly over the course.

Kellie Brown's Iron-Distance Bike Racing Fueling and Hydration Statistics (Approx.)

Fluid ounces consumed per hour: 24 oz.
Fluid (oz.) per hour to body weight (lbs.) ratio: 0.21

Calories per hour: 380
Calories per hour to body weight (lbs.) ratio: 3.3

Nutritional ratios: 100% carbohydrates, 0% protein, and 0% fat

---

Marathons: Kellie's plan is usually to consume energy gels with caffeine (100 calories, all carbohydrates) at miles 5, 10, 14, 18, and 22, which, based on her usual pace, means about every 40 minutes in the early stages of the race, and then every 32 minutes in the later stages. Kellie drinks water when consuming each energy gel, but consumes an energy drink at all other aid stations. Estimating a total of twelve aid stations and 6 ounces per aid station (at seven of which she consumes an energy drink, and at five of which she consumes water), Kellie consumes approximately 72 ounces of fluid containing about 315 calories (all carbohydrates).

Kellie Brown's Marathon Racing Fueling and Hydration Statistics (Approx.)

Fluid ounces consumed per hour: 21 oz.
Fluid (oz.) per hour to body weight (lbs.) ratio: 0.18

Calories per hour: 235
Calories per hour to body weight (lbs.) ratio: 2.0

Nutritional ratios: 100% carbohydrates, 0% protein, and 0% fat

---

Kellie Brown's Pre-Training Fueling and Hydration Routine

Before her regular early-morning training sessions of 60 minutes or less, Kellie drinks about 12 ounces of Gatorade (90 calories, all carbohydrates). If the session is in excess of 60 minutes, or it calls for a higher level of intensity, Kellie may also have either a banana (120 calories; about 97% carbohydrates and 3% protein) or one slice of whole-wheat bread with 2 to 3 teaspoons of peanut butter (300 calories; about 26% carbohydrates, 15% protein, and 59% fat). Before an afternoon or evening regular training session, Kellie will usually eat a PowerBar (240 calories; about 70% carbohydrates, 15% protein, and 15% fat) one to two hours beforehand. She will also have about 12 ounces of Gatorade (90 calories, all carbohydrates) within the hour leading up to her training session.

Kellie practices her exact pre-race fueling and hydration plan before all of her longer training sessions throughout the year. Kellie finds that this has made her race-day fueling and hydration routine very efficient and reliable.

Kellie Brown's Post-Training Fueling and Hydration Routine

Immediately following most regular training sessions, Kellie will have 8 ounces of Muscle Milk (150 calories; about 24% carbohydrates, 52% protein, and 24% fat), plus possible additional energy drinks and water. For longer training sessions of two and a half hours or more, Kellie typically doubles this amount.

3. Endurance Athlete: Scott Gac

Scott Gac has raced competitively for more than ten years. He focuses primarily on all triathlon distances up to the Iron-distance, and all road-racing distances up to the full marathon. Among his many accomplishments, Scott has qualified for and competed in the ITU Long Distance World Championships, the Hawaii Ironman World Championships, and the Boston Marathon multiple times. The most interesting feature of Scott's pre-race and race fueling and hydration routines is that they are 100 percent liquid. Unable to properly digest solid food on race day, probably due to pre-race pressure, Scott finds liquid sources work best for him. Scott is 6 feet tall, and he races at about 158 pounds.

Scott Gac's Pre-Race Fueling and Hydration Routine

For all races Scott wakes up at least three hours before the start and consumes three 8-ounce bottles of Ensure nutrition drink (750 calories; about 65% carbohydrates, 14% protein, and 21% fat). Scott then gradually consumes two 20-ounce bottles of energy drink (300 calories, all carbohydrates) over the next three hours, and then has one energy gel (100 calories, all carbohydrates) just before the race start.

Scott Gac's Pre-Race Fueling and Hydration Statistics (Approx.)

Fluid ounces consumed: 64 oz.
Fluid (oz.) to body weight (lbs.) ratio: 0.41

Calories consumed: 1,150
Calories to body weight (lbs.) ratio: 7.3

Nutritional ratios: 77% carbohydrates, 9% protein, and 14% fat

---

Scott Gac's Race Fueling and Hydration Routine

For long-course triathlon events, Scott consumes an energy gel (100 calories, all carbohydrates) every 45 minutes, and 32 to 36 ounces of sports drink per hour (240 to 270 calories per hour, all carbohydrates), from the time he gets on the bike until the time he crosses the finish line. His totals are 32 to 36 ounces of fluid per hour, and 373 to 403 calories per hour. For running events, Scott's routine is much the same, but since it's sometimes difficult to consume this much fluid per hour while running, he finds that he usually consumes a little less than his 32- to 36-ounce target.

Scott Gac's Race Fueling and Hydration Statistics (Approx.)

Fluid ounces consumed per hour: 32 to 36 oz.
Fluid oz. per hour as a percentage of body weight (lbs.): 0.22

Calories per hour: 373 to 403
Calories per hour to body weight (lbs.) ratio: 2.5

Nutritional ratios: 100% carbohydrates, 0% protein, and 0% fat

---

Scott Gac's Pre-Training Fueling and Hydration Routine

Scott usually consumes 16 to 20 ounces of water before shorter running sessions, and 16 to 20 ounces of energy drink for longer sessions over 75 minutes. He finds solid foods don't sit well with him before running, so he sticks with liquids. For swimming and cycling, however, Scott will often have either a baked sweet potato or a banana and a homemade muffin.

Scott Gac's Post-Training Fueling and Hydration Routine

Scott typically has fruit (e.g., banana, apple, or orange) and a small quantity of protein (e.g., boiled egg, canned chicken, tablespoon of peanut butter, etc.) within 45 minutes after training. While typically this will total about 300 calories, he may have more than 300 calories after longer sessions. Scott will also typically consume another 20 to 30 ounces of water within 45 minutes after his training sessions.

4. Endurance Athlete: Peter Hyland

Peter Hyland has been an elite endurance athlete for more than ten years, and he has won or placed in his age group at competitions all over the world. Peter focuses on all triathlon distances up to the full Iron-distance, and all road-racing distances up to the marathon. Peter's many accomplishments include being a sub 2:50 marathoner and qualifying for and racing in the Ironman World Championships in Kona, Hawaii. Peter is 6 feet tall and races at about 160 pounds.

Peter Hyland's Pre-Race Fueling and Hydration Routine

For Iron-distance events, Peter wakes up two and half to three hours before the start time and immediately consumes one large blueberry bagel (322 calories; 80% carbohydrates, 14% protein, and 6% fat), a banana (105 calories; 96% carbohydrates, 4% protein, and 0% fat), and one PowerBar (240 calories; 70% carbohydrates, 15 % protein, and 15% fat). He also begins drinking a 32-ounce bottle of Gatorade (200 calories, all carbohydrates). After arriving at the race site, he has usually completed his first bottle of Gatorade, and he will begin a second bottle. He continues to gradually drink this second bottle right up to about 20 minutes before the race. Peter tries to consume as much of this second bottle as possible, but sometimes only completes about half to three-quarters of it (100 to 150 calories, all carbohydrates). Finally, about 20 minutes before the start of the race, Peter has half of a PowerBar (120 calories; 70% carbohydrates, 15% protein, and 15% fat).

Peter Hyland's Pre-Race Fueling and Hydration Statistics (Approx.)

Fluid ounces consumed: 48 to 56 oz.
Fluid (oz.) to body weight (lbs.) ratio: 0.30 to 0.35

Calories consumed: 1,087 to 1,137
Calories to body weight (lbs.) ratio: 6.8 to 7.2

Nutritional ratios: 84% carbohydrates, 10% protein, and 6% fat

---

Peter Hyland's Race Fueling and Hydration Routine

For the bike portion of half and full Iron-distance events, Peter waits about 15 minutes to settle in after the swim and then begins drinking Gatorade at a rate of 24 to 32 ounces per hour (150 to 200 calories, all carbohydrates). He starts with two bottles on his bike, and once they have been completed, he switches to whatever energy drink is being offered on the course. During the bike, Peter also has either a pre-cut half of a PowerBar (120 calories; 70% carbohydrates, 15% protein, and 15% fat) or an energy gel (100 calories, all carbohydrates), alternating every 50 minutes (120 to 144 calories per hour). For the run segment, Peter tries to maintain the exact same fluid and calorie intake. However, he switches from an alternating mix of energy gels and half PowerBars to energy gels only.

Peter Hyland's Race Fueling and Hydration Statistics (Approx.)

Fluid ounces consumed per hour: 24 to 32 oz.
Fluid (oz.) per hour to body weight (lbs.) ratio: 0.15 to 0.20

Calories per hour: 270 to 344
Calories per hour to body weight (lbs.) ratio: 1.7 to 2.2

Nutritional ratios: 93% carbohydrates, 5% protein; and 2% fat

---

Peter Hyland's Pre-Training Fueling and Hydration Routine

Peter's pre-training fueling varies depending on the time of day, which can be either early morning, early afternoon, late afternoon, or evening. Most often Peter will consume Gatorade and half of a bagel—relatively light fueling, but rich in carbohydrates.

Peter Hyland's Post-Training Fueling and Hydration Routine

Peter's post-training fueling also varies due to the fact that he trains at several different times throughout the week, but for his most important sessions, which are usually his long weekend sessions, he likes to have a large bowl of oatmeal with a mashed banana, chocolate Muscle Milk (light), and a glass of regular chocolate milk, all within 30 minutes after the session. He will usually also include some additional Gatorade and water within these first 30 minutes.

5. Endurance Athlete: Dave Mantle

Dave Mantle has raced competitively for more than ten years. He focuses primarily on road races all the way up to Ultra Distance marathons, and triathlons up to the Iron-distance. Among his many accomplishments, Dave has completed the famous Marathon des Sables, which is a 156-mile ultra-marathon through the Sahara Desert in Morocco. Dave's height is 6 feet, 1 inch, and he races at about 160 pounds.

Dave Mantle's Pre-Race Fueling and Hydration Routine

Dave typically wakes up four hours before the start of the race and consumes two cups of black coffee (300 ml, or 10.1 oz.), a glass of water (300 ml, or 10.1 oz.), and one bowl of jumbo oats porridge (361 calories; about 68% carbohydrates, 12% protein, and 20% fat) mixed with water (100 ml, or 3.4 oz.), a medium banana (105 calories; about 92% carbohydrates, 4% protein, and 4% fat), and honey (60 calories, all carbohydrates). For longer races like the Iron-distance triathlon or an ultra-marathon, Dave adds to this one bagel with a small amount of peanut butter (300 calories; about 70% carbohydrates, 10% protein, and 20% fat). From this point until about 30 minutes before the start, Dave gradually drinks a bottle of PowerBar energy drink (750 ml, or 25.4 oz.; 140 calories, all carbohydrates). Then, with 30 minutes to go until the start, Dave consumes another bottle of water (100 ml, or 3.4 oz.). Finally, with 10 minutes to go, Dave has one PowerBar gel (110 calories, all carbohydrates).

Dave Mantle's Pre-Race (Over Five Hours) Fueling and Hydration Statistics (Approx.)

Fluid ounces consumed: 52 oz. (1,550 ml)
Fluid (oz.) to body weight (lbs.) ratio: 0.33

Calories consumed: 1,076 (ultras and Iron-distance); 776 (shorter events)
Calories to body weight (lbs.) ratio: 6.7 (ultras and Iron-distance); 4.9 (shorter events)

Nutritional ratios: 82% carbohydrates, 6% protein, and 12% fat

---

Dave Mantle's Race Fueling and Hydration Routine

From the time the gun goes off for an ultra-marathon, or from the time the bike portion begins for an Iron-distance triathlon, Dave consumes one energy gel (100 calories, all carbohydrates) every 25 minutes, and he completes an energy drink (750 ml, or 25.4 oz.) every 45 minutes (140 calories, all carbohydrates). This equates to about 1,000 milliliters (33.8 oz.) of fluid and 460 calories per hour. For races over ten hours, Dave will often switch from energy drink to cola after the ten-hour mark, usually three cups per hour (about 300 calories, all carbohydrates). Dave may also switch from energy gels to half-bananas in the later stages of these very long races.

Dave Mantle's Race Fueling and Hydration Statistics (Approx.)

Fluid ounces consumed per hour: 33.8 oz. (1.0 liter)
Fluid (oz.) per hour to body weight (lbs.) ratio: 0.21

Calories per hour: 460
Calories per hour to body weight (lbs.) ratio: 2.9

Nutritional ratios: 100% carbohydrates, 0% protein, and 0% fat

---

Dave Mantle's Pre-Training Fueling and Hydration Routine

Dave has black coffee (250 ml, or 8.5 oz.) just before he begins most training sessions. If the session is less than 75 minutes long, he drinks water (650 ml, or 22 oz.) with a Nuun electrolyte tablet. Dave takes an energy gel with him during these shorter sessions, just in case he experiences low energy, but finds that he rarely needs it. For longer sessions of 75 minutes or more, which are usually on weekend mornings, Dave has 500 milliliters of coffee and a bowl of oatmeal with a banana and water, two hours before the start. Dave then has an energy gel with water (about 300 ml, or 10.1 oz.) 10 minutes before beginning the session.

Dave Mantle's Post-Training Fueling and Hydration Routine

For any sessions that are in excess of 75 minutes and/or include higher-intensity work, Dave has a carbohydrate-and-protein recovery drink within

20 minutes of completing the workout. The one he likes best comes in powder form that is mixed with water (400 ml, or 13.5 oz.) and has 400 calories. The ratio of carbs to protein is about 3 to 1.

6. Endurance Athlete: Russ O'Hara

Russ O'Hara has been an elite endurance athlete for more than ten years, and he has won or placed in his age group at competitions all over the world. Russ focuses on all triathlon distances up to the full Iron-distance, and all road-racing distances up to the marathon. Among his many accomplishments, Russ has qualified for and raced in the Ironman 70.3 World Championships. Russ is 5 feet, 11 inches tall, and races at about 180 pounds.

Russ O'Hara's Pre-Race Fueling and Hydration Routine

Russ wakes up three hours before the start and consumes a bagel with Nutella (354 calories; 66% carbohydrates, 16% protein, and 8% fat); two Winners energy bars (368 calories; 75% carbohydrates, 11% protein, and 13% fat.); and "Evolve AI" energy drink (750 ml, or 25.4 oz.; 315 calories; 60% carbohydrates, 38% protein, and 2% fat.). Russ then gradually sips 750 milliliters (25.4 oz.) of water right up until the time of the race. Then, 30 minutes before the start, Russ consumes one Enervit energy gel (120 calories, all carbohydrates).

Russ O'Hara's Pre-Race Fueling and Hydration Statistics (Approx.)

Fluid ounces consumed: 1.5 liters (50.7 oz.)
Fluid (oz.) to body weight (lbs.) ratio: 0.28

Calories consumed: 1,157
Calories to body weight (lbs.) ratio: 6.4

Nutritional ratios: 72% carbohydrates, 18% protein, and 10% fat

---

Russ O'Hara's Race Fueling and Hydration Routine

As soon as Russ settles in on the Iron-distance bike leg, he begins taking one Enervit energy gel (120 calories; all carbohydrates) every 25 minutes, and continues this pattern right through to the finish of the run. Russ also starts the bike with two 750-milliliter (25.4 oz.) bottles of "Evolve AI" energy drink (315 calories; 60% carbohydrates, 38% protein, and 2% fat), and completes one every 35 minutes. Once these two bottles have been completed, Russ begins to take additional bottles of energy drink from the aid stations and continues to consume one every 35 minutes. Depending on the race, these additional 750-milliliter (25.4 oz.) bottles of energy drink are likely to have about 150 calories each, all of which are carbohydrates. Russ always practices with the race's energy drink during his longer training sessions leading up to the races, so he is sure that his body will be used to it. For extra sodium, Russ also has two salt-stick caps with a small amount of water every hour. Once onto the run course, Russ usually stays with the same routine. However, he sometimes switches over from energy drinks to cola if he feels he needs a change.

Russ O'Hara's Race Fueling and Hydration Statistics (Approx.)

Fluid ounces consumed per hour: 1.28 liters (43.5 oz.)
Fluid (oz.) per hour to body weight (lbs.) ratio: 0.24

Calories per hour: 537 (Note: Average after first 70 minutes on the bike.)
Calories per hour to body weight (lbs.) ratio: 2.9

Nutritional ratios: 100% carbohydrates, 0% protein, and 0% fat

(Note: This is after the first 70 minutes on the bike, during which Russ consumes additional protein and fat from his energy drinks.)

Russ O'Hara's Pre-Training Fueling and Hydration Routine

Russ practices his exact pre-race fueling before all of his longer training sessions. For other shorter sessions, Russ will usually have a bowl of rice porridge with apple, raisins, and banana with almond milk (330 calories; 70% carbohydrates, 10% protein, and 20% fat.), 750 milliliters (25.4 oz.) of "Evolve AI" energy drink (315 calories; 60% carbohydrates, 38% protein, and 2% fat), and 500 milliliters (17 oz.) of water.

Russ O'Hara's Post-Training Fueling and Hydration Routine

Russ consumes a blend of 750 milliliters (25.4 oz.) of "Evolve 3 Whey" recovery drink (160 calories; 7% carbohydrates, 81% protein, and 12% fat) with fresh berries and water.

7. Endurance Athlete: Greg Perangelo

Greg Perangelo has raced competitively for only a few years but has accomplished a great deal in that time. He focuses on all triathlon distances up to the full Iron-distance, and all road-racing distances up to the marathon. Among his many accomplishments, Greg frequently wins or places in his age group at all distances, and he has qualified and raced the Boston Marathon. Greg's height is 5 feet, 11 inches, and he races at about 165 pounds.

Greg Perangelo's Pre-Race Fueling and Hydration Routine

For all races Greg wakes up at least three hours before the start and consumes three PowerBars (720 calories; about 70% carbohydrates, 15% protein, and 15% fat), 8 to 12 ounces of coffee, 8 to 12 ounces of water, and 24 ounces of GU Electrolyte Brew energy drink (150 calories, all carbohydrates). He then consumes another 24 ounces of GU Electrolyte Brew energy drink about one hour before the swim start, as well as a GU Roctane energy gel (100 calories, all carbohydrates) about 10 minutes before the swim start.

Greg Perangelo's Pre-Race Fueling and Hydration Statistics (Approx.)

Fluid ounces consumed: 64 to 72 oz.
Fluid (oz.) to body weight (lbs.) ratio: 0.39 to 0.43

Calories consumed: 1,120
Calories to body weight (lbs.) ratio: 6.8

Nutritional ratios: 80% carbohydrates, 10% protein, and 10% fat

---

Greg Perangelo's Race Fueling and Hydration Routine

For longer events like the Iron-distance triathlon, Greg begins on the bike by consuming one Roctane energy gel (100 calories, all carbohydrates) every 30 minutes, and 24 ounces of GU Electrolyte Brew (150 calories, all carbohydrates) energy drink every 45 to 50 minutes. Greg targets these same amounts on the run. However, he usually switches his hydration to whatever energy drink the race is offering, and he does his best to estimate his fluid amounts while drinking it from cups at each aid station.

Greg Perangelo's Race Fueling and Hydration Statistics (Approx.)

Fluid ounces consumed per hour: 29 to 32 oz.
Fluid (oz.) per hour to body weight (lbs.) ratio: 0.19

Calories per hour: 380 to 400
Calories per hour to body weight (lbs.) ratio: 2.4

Nutritional ratios: 100% carbohydrates, 0% protein, and 0% fat

---

Greg Perangelo's Pre-Training Fueling and Hydration Routine

Greg does most of his training first thing in the early morning before work, and he typically sticks to the same proven routine. He has a bowl of oatmeal with walnuts, raisins, and blueberries mixed with soy milk (670 calories; about 60% carbohydrates, 7% protein, and 33% fat), about 8 ounces of water, and a cup of coffee (8 ounces).

Greg Perangelo's Post-Training Fueling and Hydration Routine

Immediately after all training sessions, Greg consumes 16 to 20 ounces of Recoverite recovery drink. The ratio of carbs to protein is about 3 to 1. Greg finds that this helps to jump-start his recovery and prepare him to feel his best before his next training session.

8. Endurance Athlete: Peter Turek

Peter Turek has been an elite age group triathlete for more than ten years. He has won his age group at major races, from short-course to Iron-distance all over the world. Peter has qualified and raced the Hawaii Ironman as well as the World Championships at virtually all distances. Peter is 5 feet, 10 inches tall and races at about 165 pounds.

Peter Turek's Pre-Race Fueling and Hydration Routine

On race-day morning, Peter wakes up three hours prior to the race start and has 12 ounces of coffee and a bowl of oatmeal with honey, peanut butter, flaxseed, and chia seeds (445 calories; about 53% carbohydrates, 36% fat, and 11% protein). Over the next two hours, Peter gradually consumes one 20-ounce bottle of Gatorade (150 calories, all carbohydrates). Then, with one hour to go prior to the start, Peter has one PowerBar (240 calories; about 70% carbohydrates, 15% fat, and 15% protein) and gradually consumes a 20-ounce bottle of water. Finally, with 10 minutes to go, Peter has one caffeinated energy gel (100 calories, all carbohydrates) for a half Iron-distance, or two caffeinated energy gels (200 calories, all carbohydrates) if it is a full Iron-distance triathlon. (Note: If it is an especially hot day, Peter will often add up to 12 ounces of fluids to the above, and, conversely, if it is an especially cool day, he may consume up to 12 ounces less.)

Peter Turek's Pre-Race Fueling and Hydration Statistics (Approx.)

Fluid ounces consumed: 52 oz.
Fluid (oz.) to body weight (lbs.) ratio: 0.32

Calories consumed: 1,035 (full Iron-distance)
Calories to body weight (lbs.) ratio: 6.3

Nutritional ratios: 72% carbohydrates, 8% protein, and 20% fat

---

Peter Turek's Race Fueling and Hydration Routine

For longer events like the Iron-distance triathlon, Peter begins on the bike by consuming one PowerBar energy gel (110 calories, all carbohydrates) every 30 minutes and 24 ounces of PowerBar Perform (210 calories, all carbohydrates) energy drink every 60 minutes. (During hot-weather races, he'll drink up to an additional 8 ounces of water per hour.) Peter targets these same amounts on the run. However, he usually switches his hydration to a combination of energy drinks (whatever is offered), gels, and water, and he does his best to estimate his fluid amounts while drinking from cups at each aid station. Since the run aid stations are normally spaced at 1-mile intervals, he alternates between energy drink only, and gel with water, at odd and even mile markers, respectively.

Peter Turek's Race Fueling and Hydration Statistics (Approx.)

Fluid ounces consumed per hour: 24 to 32 oz.
Fluid (oz.) per hour to body weight (lbs.) ratio: 0.15 to 0.19

Calories per hour: 430
Calories per hour to body weight (lbs.) ratio: 2.6

Nutritional ratios: 100% carbohydrates, 0% protein, 0% fat

Peter Turek's Pre-Training Fueling and Hydration Routine

During the weekdays, Peter will split his training into two sessions (morning versus evening); swim and strength in the morning, bike and run in the evening. Training on the weekends usually includes a long "brick session" (i.e., bike ride followed by a run) and long run, both of which are usually done early in the morning. Most mornings, he has a bowl (1 cup) of multigrain cereal, with (1% fat) milk (260 calories; about 75% carbohydrates, 15% fat, and 10% protein), and an 8-ounce cup of coffee. Just prior to his afternoon workouts, he will consume a Clif Bar (240 calories) with 8 ounces of water. Training sessions (bike and/or run) that last up to 60 minutes are done with water only, between 60 and 120 minutes with Accelerade (24 oz. per hour), and in sessions of more than 120 minutes, Peter utilizes his same hydration and fueling race strategy presented above.

Peter Turek's Post-Training Fueling and Hydration Routine

Immediately following his longer (two hours-plus) training sessions, Peter will consume a serving (12 oz.) of Endurox R4 (270 calories; about 77%

carbohydrates, 4% fat, and 19% protein), followed by a full meal (lunch or dinner). He prefers to eat foods that are high in protein (legumes) and good fat (omega-3s), such as salmon and flaxseed.

We hope the above plans will be helpful in determining the optimal plan for you. We are all different when it comes to fueling and hydration, so we need to test and fine-tune our plans in training to discover what works best for us. Our suggestion is to select the plan (or plans) in this chapter that best fits your situation. Then, practice it and make adjustments as needed in your longer training sessions. Once you have determined your own unique plan, don't put it away on a shelf and forget about it. Continue to practice it year-round in at least one long session per week and make it second nature.

CHAPTER 9

Make IronFit Strength Training and Nutrition Work for You

Only the weak attempts to accomplish what
he knows he can already achieve.

—*Stella Juarez*

W e have covered a great deal of information in this book. The key now is to take from this book the programs and tools that best fit you as an athlete—for your particular races and goals—and put them to work for you. To help you do this, we will present three athlete examples: Heidi Harrier, Karl Kona, and Ralph Rookie. These fictitious athletes are composites of actual athletes with whom we have worked over the years. We will take a look at each athlete's specific profile and then not only select the best programs and routines for each, but also show exactly when and where to build them into their overall training and racing plan.

Example One: Heidi Harrier

Athlete Profile: Heidi Harrier is forty-one years old (5 feet, 6 inches tall, 125 pounds) and will be racing the New York City Marathon in early November, which is about sixteen weeks away. Heidi has been competing in road races in the 5K to marathon range for several years, and this will be her fifth marathon. Her goal for the New York City Marathon is not only to better her personal best marathon time of 3:51, but also to qualify for the Boston Marathon by finishing under the qualifying standard of 3:45. She is following one of the marathon training plans in our book *Mastering the Marathon*, which includes five days of running and two days of cross-training per week, and she plans to include a greater focus on strength training and nutrition than she has in the past, to improve her chances of achieving her goals.

Warm-up and Flexibility Program: Heidi used the Easy Eight warm-up routine (Chapter 2, page 12) before all her runs, cross-training, and strength-training sessions. Once she became proficient at it, the routine only took her about 5 minutes to complete. She found that it made her feel better prepared for each session, and her actual training performance improved as a result. Most importantly, for the first time, she experienced no injuries while preparing for this marathon, and she felt her new focus on a proper warm-up contributed to her health.

Mental Preparation Program: In addition to preparing her body with the Easy Eight, Heidi prepared herself mentally with the visualization approach, "Been There, Done That" (Chapter 2, page 20). Because of her tight schedule, she could not always squeeze in the time for visualizations, but she always tried to include her routine before at least the three most important runs of the week in her program. Heidi usually ran first thing in the morning, and she found that she really enjoyed the centered feeling she achieved from preparing with visualization in the calm, quiet mornings.

Strength and Core Training Program: Heidi completed the Runners—Road Racer (5K to Full Marathon) functional strength-training program (Chapter 3, page 59) two times per week. She included it after her runs on Monday and Friday. Of her training plan's five weekly runs per week, Monday's and Friday's runs were the shortest and at a moderate intensity level, so not only did these runs help to warm her up for strength training, but her energy level was also higher after these two workouts than it was after the three other, more-challenging runs in the weekly plan. She progressed through all three cycles of the Runners—Road Racer Program (Off-Season, Preseason, and Competitive Season), and as she mastered each exercise, she moved up from the Basic level to the Intermediate progression, and then to the Advanced progression, as suggested in the program. Heidi had never stuck with a strength-training program before in a marathon training cycle, but found that even when starting with the Easy Eight warm-up routine, she was able to complete the Off-Season version of the program in less than 30 minutes, and the Preseason and Competitive-Season versions in less than 25 minutes. The program remained doable even when her running durations increased and required more time.

General Healthy Eating Plan

Heidi chose to use a six-meals-a-day approach because she found it kept her energy level high and consistent throughout the day. Using the "14 calories per pound" approach, she determined that her Active BMR was about 1,750 calories per day, so she patterned her regular diet on the "Plan 1750" Seven-Day Eating Plan (Chapter 5, page 168). Since she did not desire to lose any weight, she made daily adjustments to this plan as needed to account for the calories utilized in training. She used www.myfitnesspal.com to track her daily calorie intake, and to help her make the necessary adjustments to keep her close to her 1,750 net calories per day target.

Fueling and Hydration Plans

- *Pre-Run:* Heidi made sure that she woke up at least 45 minutes before her morning runs so that she had time to fuel and hydrate well before her sessions. After testing and practicing with various options over a couple of months, Heidi determined her optimal plan to be the following: She would have a balanced energy bar (230 calories), water (8 oz.), and coffee (8 oz.) soon after waking. Then, while dressing for her run and while completing her warm-up program and mental preparation, she gradually sipped 8 ounces of energy drink (72 calories). Her totals before her runs were 24 ounces and about 302 calories (80% carbohydrates, 10% fats, and 10% protein).
- *Run:* Four of Heidi's five runs per week were less than 75 minutes, so she hydrated with straight water for the entire run (Chapter 6, page 210). She used the Sweat Rate Test (Chapter 6, page 198) to determine that her hydration needs are about 20 ounces per hour, and she therefore carried this amount in her hydration belt. During her one run of the week that was longer than 75 minutes, she practiced and perfected her exact race fueling and hydration program (see "Race" below).
- *Post-Run:* Heidi always took advantage of the "45-minute window" after each run to get a jump start on replenishing her stored carbohydrates (glycogen) levels (Chapter 7, page 215). By doing so, she found that her energy level was considerably higher for her next training session. Typically, Heidi would either have a recovery drink (which included carbohydrates, protein, and fats), or she would have an additional energy drink and a balanced energy bar (which included carbohydrates, protein, and fats).

- *Race:* Heidi's simple routine, which was similar to what many of the eight profiled athletes used in Chapter 8, included only energy drink and energy gels. She determined in advance from the race website what energy drink would be offered during the race, and then she practiced with that energy drink in all of her longer runs. She also practiced drinking from cups, as she planned to get her hydration from the aid stations during the race. Since she requires about 20 ounces of fluid per hour, as determined by the Sweat Rate Test (Chapter 6, page 198), she tried to get as close as possible to this amount. Since her target time of 3:45 indicated that she would need to consume about 75 ounces of fluid during the race (i.e., 3.75 hours x 20 ounces = 75 ounces), and since she planned to utilize twelve aid stations on the course, she tried to consume a little more than 6 ounces at each aid station (i.e., 75 ounces / 12 aid stations = 6.25 ounces per aid station). Heidi also consumed a GU energy gel (100 calories), which she carried in a back pocket, every 40 minutes during the race. This equates to five gels for the entire race. Heidi's total calories consumed during the race were approximately 1,063 (563 from energy drinks and 500 from GU), or approximately 283 calories per hour (i.e., 1,063 calories / 3.75 hours = 283.5 calories per hour).

Heidi's Results: Heidi had her most productive and rewarding marathon preparation phase ever. She arrived at her race healthy, mentally focused, and feeling stronger than ever. While maintaining her target weight throughout the training process, Heidi was thrilled to learn that her body-fat ratios had actually improved due to her focus on strength training and nutrition. Her body fat, which was at an already acceptable 18 percent before this training phase, was now down to 15 percent. Heidi raced an evenly paced race, but after 20 miles realized that she felt surprisingly strong and picked her pace up a bit over the final 10K. She exceeded her goals with a personal record time of 3:42, which was comfortably under the Boston Marathon qualifying time of 3:45. Look for Heidi in Boston on the third Monday in April!

Example Two: Karl Kona

Athlete Profile: Karl Kona is thirty-five years old (5 feet, 11 inches tall, 180 pounds) and will be racing Ironman Florida in early November, about eight months from this starting point. Karl has been competing in triathlons for three years, but this will be his first Iron-distance triathlon. While he knows that it's usually not recommended to have a time goal in your first Iron-distance triathlon, Karl feels that based on his times at shorter distances, he would like to break twelve hours. He plans on following one of the Iron-distance training plans in the book *Be Iron Fit, 2nd Edition,* and to include a greater focus on strength training and nutrition than he has in the past in order to improve his chances of achieving his goals.

Warm-up and Flexibility Program: Karl used the Easy Eight warm-up routine (Chapter 2, page 12) at least three times per week. His masters swim group meets on Monday, Wednesday, and Thursday mornings, and he used the program before all of these sessions to prepare his body to perform at its best. Karl had hoped to complete this warm-up and flexibility program before his other sessions, as well, but due to a tight schedule and the fact that none of the other sessions were first thing in the morning, he usually chose to let it slip on some of the other days.

Mental Preparation Program: The swim was Karl's weakest link, so he also used the breathing exercise (Chapter 2, page 20) to help get more dialed in both mentally and physically before his workouts in this sport. Since swimming is such a technique-oriented sport, Karl was hoping that this mental approach would help him to relax more in the water and break through to new levels of performance in this sport.

Strength and Core Training Program: Karl completed the Long-Course Triathlete Functional Strength-Training Program (Chapter 3, page 32) two times per week. He included it on Wednesdays and Sundays. Those days worked best for two reasons: First, Karl found that trying to complete his strength and core training on a swim day was not optimal. Either his arms were too tired from swimming first to have a productive strength and core session, or his arms were too tired from strength and core training to have a productive swim session. Second, Wednesdays and Sundays are days he usually has more-moderate bike and run sessions planned, which helped him to feel more rested and warmed up for his strength and core sessions.

He progressed through all three cycles of this functional strength and core program (Off-Season, Preseason, and Competitive Season), and as he mastered each exercise, he moved up to the higher progressions of each exercise as outlined in the program. Karl found that he could complete the program in less than 25 minutes in the Off-Season, and in less than 20 minutes in the Preseason and Competitive Season. He was able to stick with it for the entire year, which he had never been able to do before. Note that Karl did not use the Easy Eight before his strength-training sessions, while he did use it before his swims.

Special Travel Program: Karl does a fair amount of traveling with his job, but by planning ahead to make sure that he had suitable training facilities and enough time to complete his planned workouts, he missed only four planned workouts due to traveling over the thirty-week training period. On those four occasions, he substituted the Special Travel Program (Chapter 3, page 132) and was very pleased with the results. Not only did he feel better mentally because he was able to squeeze in a good strength-training session, but he also found that he actually enjoyed the change of pace.

General Healthy Eating Plan: Karl planned to use a six-meals-a-day approach because he found it kept his energy level high and consistent throughout the day. Using the formulas in Chapter 4, he determined that his Active BMR was about 2,500 calories per day, so he patterned his regular diet on the Plan 2500 Seven-Day Eating Plan (Chapter 5, page 189). Since he did not desire to lose any weight, he made adjustments to this plan to account for the calories utilized in training. He used a daily worksheet to track his daily calorie intake and to help him make the necessary adjustments to remain close to his 2,500 net calories per day target.

Fueling and Hydration Plans

- *Pre-Training:* Karl had never fueled and hydrated before his three weekly early-morning swim sessions in years past, so he wisely started with a light program and then gradually built on it over time. He found that pre-training fueling and hydration gave him much higher levels of energy, which was especially important, since the swim was where he most needed to focus. He would wake up an hour before the start of his swim session and have a balanced energy bar

(250 calories), water (12 oz.), and coffee (8 oz.) soon after waking. Then, while dressing for his swim and while completing his warm-up program and mental preparation, he gradually sipped 20 ounces of energy drink (150 calories). He would save a little of the energy drink for the short drive to the pool, to help wash down the GU energy gel with caffeine that he would consume about 10 minutes before he entered the pool. His pre-swim totals were typically about 40 ounces of fluid and about 500 calories (86% carbohydrates, 7% fats, and 7% protein).

Karl used the exact same pre-training fueling and hydration approach for Saturdays and Sundays, since both days started with an early workout. On Saturdays it was a long bike, and on Sundays it was a long run, but all other workouts during the week occurred later in the day at a point when he had already consumed significant calories and hydration. For these sessions, Karl would simply consume about 20 ounces of energy drink and a GU energy gel about 30 minutes before heading out the door.

Over the course of his thirty-week training program, Karl gradually increased the amounts in his Saturday morning pre-training fueling and hydration routine and began to start it earlier and earlier to better simulate the three preparatory hours he would have on his actual race-day morning. To the amounts above he gradually added a second balanced energy bar and an additional 24 ounces of energy drink. This raised his totals to about 64 ounces and 1,000 calories. He reached these levels about eight weeks before his Iron-distance triathlon and then repeated it every Saturday right up until his race. This then became the exact routine that he followed on race-day morning.

- *Training:* Of the ten separate weekly workouts in Karl's thirty-week plan, eight were of 75 minutes or less in duration, so Karl consumed straight water all of the way for these (Chapter 7, page 210), based on the amount determined in his Sweat Rate Test (Chapter 6, page 198), which was 30 ounces per hour. Karl of course carried his fluids in bike bottles for his cycling sessions, but since most of his runs were on the treadmill, he used a bike bottle for them as well. During his two longer workouts of the week, Karl practiced and perfected his exact race fueling and hydration program (see "Race" below).

- *Post-Training:* Karl planned ahead to make sure that he took advantage of the "45-minute window" after all sessions to get a jump start on replenishing his stored carbohydrate (glycogen) levels (Chapter 7, page 215). This included always having balanced energy bars, energy drinks, or recovery drinks in his car, so they would be available for him after swimming, and for any other training sessions to which he drove. With ten workouts per week, this helped Karl immensely to recover quickly and to keep his energy level high.
- *Race:* Karl studied the routines of the accomplished Iron-distance triathletes in Chapter 8, tested some of their approaches in training, and arrived at a program that included energy drinks and energy gels. He found out from the race what energy drink they would be using on the course and he trained with it for all of his Saturday long bikes and Sunday long runs. He also practiced drinking from cups during one run per week during the last few weeks before his race, to perfect his technique.

  Since he requires about 30 ounces of fluid per hour, as determined by the Sweat Rate Test (Chapter 6, page 198), he tried to get as close as possible to this amount. This would equate to completing a 20-ounce bottle of energy drink about every 40 minutes on the bike, and then drinking an equivalent amount from cups on the run. Karl carried his energy gels in a bento box on the bike and in the back webbed pocket of his tri-suit on the run.

  With an expected bike time of about six hours, Karl planned to consume nine 20-ounce bike bottles (360 minutes to complete bike portion / 40 minutes to complete each 20-ounce bottle = 9 bottles). Karl carried the first three bottles on his bike and then took bottles 4 through 9 from the aid stations (which were spaced 10 miles apart). Karl carried fourteen energy gels (100 calories each) in the bento box on his bike and consumed one every 25 minutes. Karl's totals for the six-hour bike were about 180 ounces and 2,750 calories (9 bottles @ 150 calories each and 14 energy gels @ 100 calories each), and 30 ounces per hour and 458 calories per hour.

  With an expected run time of 4.5 hours, Karl expected to consume 135 ounces of energy drink (4.5 hours x 30 ounces per hour = 135 ounces). With twenty-five aid stations on the run course, Karl tried to consume 5 to 6 ounces at each aid station (135 ounces / 25 aid stations = 5.4 ounces). In addition, Karl planned to consume a 100-calorie energy gel every 30 minutes on the run. Karl's totals for the four-and-a-half-hour run were about 135 ounces and 1,912.5 calories (135 ounces = 1,012.5 calories; 9 energy gels = 900 calories; 1,012.5 + 900 = 1,912.5) and 30 ounces and 425 calories per hour (1,912.5 calories / 4.5 hours = 425 calories per hour).

Karl's Results: Karl had what he described as one of the most rewarding experiences of his life. Not only did he exceed his goal, but he also thoroughly enjoyed the entire nine-month journey. Karl arrived in Florida in November feeling healthy, mentally focused, and in the best form of his life. His weight was down to 172 pounds, which he wasn't really trying to do, but he sure liked the results, as his body-fat ratios had greatly improved due to his focus on strength training and nutrition. His body fat, which was at an already very good 13 percent before this training phase, was now down to a very impressive 10 percent. Karl's time of 11:32 was well ahead of his expectations, and he is now more excited than ever to see what he is capable of in this sport. Karl plans on targeting another Iron-distance triathlon next year with the goal of breaking eleven hours. His long-term goal now is to someday race at the Ironman World Championships in Kona, Hawaii.

Example Three: Ralph Rookie

Athlete Profile: Ralph Rookie is forty-nine years old (5 feet, 8 inches tall, 240 pounds) and has set the goal of completing a local half-marathon race to celebrate his fiftieth birthday in about ten months. Ralph has enjoyed golf for most of his adult life, but this will be his first endurance sports competition. Along with the goal of completing the half-marathon, Ralph has a second goal of weighing less than 200 pounds by the day of the race. His third and most important goal is to enjoy the process not only so that it motivates him to do more road racing, but also, so that he will embrace the endurance sports lifestyle and make it part of his fitness and health plan for life. Ralph plans to start by running for 30 minutes a day, three times per week, and then gradually to build up to five runs per week in the 45- to 60-minute range.

Ralph also plans to include strength and core training and nutrition as part of his training program.

Warm-up and Flexibility Program: Ralph used the Easy Eight warm-up routine (Chapter 2, page 12) before all of his runs. The routine took him only 5 minutes to complete, and he felt strongly that as a first-time endurance athlete, it was especially important for him to prepare his body well before each workout. Ralph was aware of how common running injuries are, and he didn't want to risk an injury spoiling his goal.

Mental Preparation Program: Ralph used the breathing and visualization approaches (Chapter 2, page 20) before most of his workouts. He found that it prepared his focus and concentration so well that he is now using the same approach to help his golf game.

Strength and Core Training Program: Ralph used the Runners—Road Racer (5K to Full Marathon) Functional Strength and Core Program (Chapter 3, page 59) two times per week. For time management reasons, he usually did it after his Monday and Wednesday runs, as he felt most warmed up and ready to go at that time. He gradually worked through the three phases (Off-Season, Preseason, and Competitive Season), as well as being able to progress from the Basic level to some of the Intermediate-level exercises.

Special Travel Program: Ralph did not need to travel much, and even when he did, he was able to get in all of his runs and strength-training sessions. He found that one of the great advantages about running is that you can pretty much do it anywhere. He also planned ahead when necessary to make sure that the hotels he'd be staying in always had a fitness center and treadmill available to him.

General Healthy Eating Plan: Ralph chose to use a six-meals-a-day approach since losing about 40 pounds was necessary to achieve his goal of weighing less than 200 pounds for his half-marathon. Through the approaches presented in Chapter 4, he determined that his Active BMR was about 3,300 net calories per day. Due to the fact that he was technically obese and had significant weight-loss goals, Ralph decided on a 10 calorie per pound daily target, instead of the "11 calories per pound" approach suggested in Chapter 4. He targeted his daily calorie target at 2,400 calories and patterned his regular diet on the Plan 2500 Seven-Day Plan (Chapter 5, page 189), with only minor adjustments to get him to 2,400 calories. He preferred to track his daily calories with www.loseit.com, suggested in Chapter 4. He used the site not only to track his calories, but also to make adjustments as needed for the calories utilized in training each day.

Fueling and Hydration Plan: After studying the approaches of several of the experienced athletes profiled in Chapter 8, Ralph decided on a simple pre-run fueling and hydration plan. Since his training sessions were almost all 75 minutes or less, he found that drinking a 20-ounce bottle of energy drink (150 calories) in the 30 minutes or so before his runs, and consuming a GU energy gel (100 calories) about 10 minutes before his runs, gave him all he needed to prepare for a great run.

Since Ralph's runs were almost all 75 minutes or less, his plan was to drink straight water. Sometimes he carried a bottle, and sometimes he ran on the treadmill with a bottle, but Ralph admitted that he skipped drinking altogether for many of his runs. He knew that this was not advised, but he felt that by hydrating well before and after his runs, he could get away with it once in a while.

Ralph's Results: Ralph not only celebrated his fiftieth birthday with a wonderful accomplishment, but he also established the foundation for many more accomplishments to come. Ralph stepped up to the starting line of his first road race ever at 194 pounds, the lightest he had been in more than twenty years. While Ralph did not have a time goal, he was very pleased with his time of 1:57 for the half-marathon, which is an average pace of a little under 9 minutes per mile. Ralph was thrilled with his accomplishment and is now motivated to race more. In fact, he is already signed up for a full marathon in six months.

Example Four: You!

Now it's your turn. Just like Heidi, Karl, and Ralph, go through each of the chapters of this book and select the plans, routines, and approaches that will best support your goals. Consider the value and importance of each element—warm-up routines, functional strength- and core-training plans, fueling and hydration routines (for pre-workout, workout, post-workout, and racing), and a healthy eating plan. Build them into your overall training strategy and commit to them. Then, consistently execute your plan. If you do, you will achieve your goals, and more. We will watch for you at the finish line!

Acknowledgments

We wish to thank the following individuals: Jonathan Beverly, M. Scott Boyles, Kellie Brown, Matthew Chiarolanzio, Debbie Debiasse, Tom Debiasse, Scott Gac, GU Energy, Yvonne Hernandez, Peter Hyland, Jeff Kellogg, Lynn Kellogg, Rick Kent, Laura Litwin, Dave Mantle, Adrianna Nelson, Russell O'Hara, Greg Perangelo, Francis Quinn, Sean Reilly, Karen Smyers, Scott Tinley, Peter Turek, Sara Vaughn, and Keith Wallman.

Glossary

Abs: Abdominal muscles.

Aerobic Energy System: An energy system that primarily utilizes oxygen and stored fat to power physical activity. This system can support activity for prolonged periods, as stored fat and oxygen are available in an almost endless supply. Even a highly trained athlete with body-fat percentages in the single digits has more than enough stored fat for several Ultra Distance races back to back.

Anaerobic Energy System: An energy system that primarily utilizes glycogen (stored sugar) to power physical activity. This system can support activity for relatively short periods of time, as the body stores sugar in relatively small quantities.

Basal Metabolic Rate (BMR): The number of calories necessary to consume each day to allow our bodies to function normally and maintain current body weight. This book also refers to "Active BMR," which is an athlete's BMR plus the additional calories needed to support normal daily activities, but not including the calories used in training and racing.

BOSU Ball (acronym for "both sides utilized"): This is an inflated "half-ball" with a flat side and a half-dome side. This popular piece of equipment is primarily used to develop balance and stability on an uneven and unstable surface.

Calorie: A calorie is a basic unit of energy. Our bodies require energy to perform virtually all functions, and our bodies get this energy in the form of calories. Carbohydrates and proteins have about 4 calories per gram, while fat has about 9 calories per gram.

Carbohydrate Loading: Various dietary approaches for the purpose of increasing glycogen stores prior to an endurance race.

Cardiovascular Drift: When an athlete's heart rate gradually increases without an increase in pace or level of performance.

Circuit Training: A method of training in which the athlete moves from one exercise to another in a series of different exercises.

Core Muscles: Includes abdominals, back, buttocks, pelvic floor, and hips.

Dumbbells: Handheld exercise weights available in various coatings from plastic to metal and various weights from one pound up to fifty-plus pounds.

Easy Eight: A 5-minute warm-up routine presented in this book that includes eight specific pre-exercise movements.

Electrolytes: Common examples of electrolytes are sodium, potassium, chloride, and carbon dioxide. Your cells need them to function properly and to keep your body's fluids in balance.

Fink Five: Five specific exercises that begin all nine of the sport-specific functional strength and core programs presented in this book.

Foam Roller: This piece of exercise equipment is made of hard foam and is usually 36 inches long and 6 inches in diameter, with varying densities used for self-myofascial release.

45-Minute Window: The time period of opportunity after a training session to jump-start the replenishment of glycogen stores.

Fueling: Within the context of endurance sports, this term refers to the process of consuming calories before, during, and after training and racing to build and maintain high levels of energy and to boost recovery.

Fueling Logistics: The means by which athletes access their needed calories during competition.

Glutes: Abbreviation for the gluteus maximus, medius, and minimus muscle group.

Glycogen: The form in which the body stores sugar (carbohydrates) for the purpose of powering muscle activity.

Hydrating: Within the context of endurance sports, this term refers to the process of drinking fluids before, during, and after training and racing to support optimal performance, safety, and good health.

Hydration Logistics: The means by which athletes access their needed fluids during competition.

Hyponatremia: An electrolyte disturbance in which sodium levels dilute well below normal. This serious medical condition can be the result of overhydration with water.

Kettle Bells: These are handheld weights, but unlike dumbbells, the center of mass is extended beyond the hand. This facilitates ballistic and swinging movements. Like dumbbells, they are available in various coatings and weights.

Medicine Ball: This is a round, weighted ball with a rubberized coating used in core and functional strength-training exercises. It is available in various weights from one to twenty pounds.

Muscle-Movement Balance: Having proportional strength in opposing muscles and proper function and coordination of muscle movement.

Overload Principle: According to the American Council on Exercise: "One of the principles of human performance that states that beneficial adaptations occur in response to demands applied to the body at levels beyond a certain threshold (overload), but within the limits of tolerance and safety."

Quads: Abbreviation for the muscles of the quadriceps.

Repetitions (Reps): The number of times an exercise movement is repeated within an exercise set.

Sarcopenia: Muscle loss related to aging.

The 75-Minute Fueling Guideline: The approximate point in a workout when water alone is not enough for most athletes to maintain the same performance level. Adequate calories, in addition to hydration, are needed.

Sets: A specific grouping of repetitions of a specific exercise movement. Typically, there will be one to three sets of each exercise within a specific exercise program.

Stability Ball (aka, Swiss Ball): This round, inflated exercise ball is the most popular and widely used piece of core-training equipment. It is important that it's properly sized to fit your height.

Stretch Cords and Resistance Tubing: These are rubber or plastic cords, usually with handles, available in various resistances.

Sweat Rate Test: A physical test performed by an athlete to help determine his or her hydration needs while training and racing.

Warm-up: A movement routine that prepares the athlete's body for training or racing by raising our core body temperature and lubricating our joints and tendons.

Suggested Reading

The books listed here have been very helpful to us over the years, providing a great deal of information as we compiled our research for this book. They may prove useful to you, as well.

Core Performance Endurance. Mark Verstegen and Pete Williams. Rodale Inc., 2007.

Core Performance: The Revolutionary Workout Program to Transform Your Body and Your Life. Mark Verstegen and Pete Williams. Rodale Inc., 2004.

The Core Program: 15 Minutes a Day that Can Change Your Life. Peggy Brill and Gerald Secor Couzens. Bantam, 2003.

Eating for Endurance. Dr. Philip Maffetone. David Barmore Productions, 1999.

Eating Well for Optimum Health. Andrew Weil, MD. Quill, 2001.

Endurance Sports Nutrition: Strategies for Training, Racing, and Recovery, 2nd Edition. Suzanne Girard Eberle, MS, RD. Human Kinetics, 2007.

Holistic Strength Training for Triathlon. Andrew Johnston. Author House, 2011.

How to Eat, Move and Be Healthy! Paul Chek. C.H.E.K. Institute Publishing, 2004.

Instant Relief: Tell Me Where It Hurts and I'll Tell You What to Do. Peggy Brill and Susan Suffes. Bantam, 2007.

Lifestyle & Weight Management Consultant Manual. Richard T. Cotton. American Council on Exercise, 1996.

Making the Cut. Jillian Michaels. Three Rivers Press, 2007.

Personal Trainer Manual: The Resource for Fitness Professionals. Richard T. Cotton, ed. American Council on Exercise, 1997.

Program Design for Personal Trainers: Bridging the Theory into Application. Douglas S. Brooks, MS. Human Kinetics, 1997.

Sports Nutrition for Endurance Athletes, 2nd Edition. Monique Ryan, MS, RD, LDN. Velo Press, 2007.

Strength Training for Triathletes. Patrick Hagerman, EdD. Velo Press, 2008.

Swiss Ball for Total Fitness. James Milligan. Barnes & Noble Books, 2005.

Training Lactate Pulse-Rate. Peter G. J. M. Janssen. Polar Electro Oy, 1987.

Tri Power: The Ultimate Strength Training, Core Conditioning, Endurance, and Flexibility Program for Triathlon Success. Paul Frediani and William Smith. Hatherleigh Press, 2007.

Understanding Nutrition, 8th Edition. Eleanor Noss Whitney and Sharon Rady Rolfes. Wadsworth Publishing Company, 1999.

Suggested Web Links

American Council on Exercise: acefitness.org

GU Energy: guenergy.com

Health Status: healthstatus.com

IronFit: ironfit.com

Live Strong: livestrong.com

Lose It: loseit.com

Lynn Kellogg, sports photographer: trilifephotos.com

Map My Run: mapmyrun.com/nutrition/calculate

My Fitness Pal: myfitnesspal.com

Perform Better: performbetter.com

United States Department of Agriculture: usda.gov

Weight Watchers: weightwatchers.com

Yvonne Hernandez, fitness model and power-lifting coach: bbasports.com

Index

weight
excuses about, 137–38
management, 147–48, 150
weight-loss, 139, 147–48
and VO2Max, 141
weight/resistance training, 9–10

weightwatchers.com, 152
women
and BMR, 147
and body fat, 140
workout productivity, 13

About the Authors

Don Fink is an internationally known triathlon and running coach/trainer and author of the popular endurance sports training books, *Be Iron Fit: Time-Efficient Training Secrets for Ultimate Fitness; Be Iron Fit, 2nd Edition;* and *Mastering the Marathon: Time-Efficient Training Secrets for the 40-plus Athlete,* all published by Lyons Press. Among his credentials, Don is a personal trainer, certified by the American Council on Exercise (ACE), and a professional member of the National Strength and Conditioning Association (NSCA). Don and his wife, Melanie, train endurance athletes on five continents through

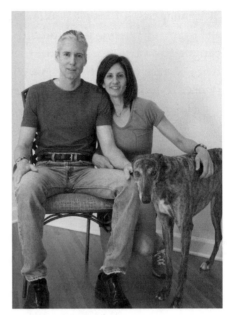

Don Fink, Melanie Fink, and Sheena
Photo by Lynn Kellogg/
www.trilifephotos.com

their business, IronFit (ironfit.com). Don and Melanie have utilized their innovative approaches to coach hundreds of athletes to personal best times and breakthrough performances in triathlon, marathon, and other sports.

In addition to being an endurance sports coach/trainer, Don Fink is also an elite athlete. He has raced more than thirty Iron-distance triathlons (2.4-mile swim, 112-mile bike, and 26.2-mile run), and has many age-group victories and course records to his credit. Don's time of 9:08 at the 2004 Ironman Florida is one of the fastest times ever recorded by an athlete in the 45–49 age group. Don Fink also placed in the top three overall in the 2002 Ultraman World Championships (6.2-mile swim, 270-mile bike, and 52.4-mile run) on the Big Island of Hawaii.

Melanie is an ACE certified personal trainer and Lifestyle and Weight Management Coach. In addition to being a sports coach/trainer and Masters

Swimming coach, Melanie Fink is also an elite athlete. She has many age-group and overall victories in triathlon and open-water swimming competitions, has completed twelve Iron-distance triathlons (including the Hawaii Ironman, twice), and she recently completed the 2010 Ultraman Canada (6.2-mile swim, 270-mile bike, and 52.4-mile run) in Penticton, British Columbia.

Don and Melanie Fink live in Morris County, New Jersey.